the hugely better
calorie
counter

carolyn humphries

D1343266

foulsham
LONDON • NEW YORK • TORONTO • SYDNEY

foulsham

Capital Point, 33 Bath Road, Slough, Berkshire
SL1 3UF, England

Foulsham books can be found in all good bookshops and direct from
www.foulsham.com

ISBN 978-0-572-03481-8

Printed and bound by CPI Group (UK) Ltd, Croydon, CR0 4YY

Contents

Introduction

There are lots of calorie counters in the bookshops, but this one is, I think, genuinely different – and hugely better. Before starting to write it, I thought very carefully about how you want to *use* a calorie counter. Having looked at those already on offer, I asked myself some questions.

- Is it useful to have to search for things under obscure brand names where you can't find them and can't compare them easily with similar products? No!

- Do you want to work out what category a food belongs to before you even try to find it? Hardly likely.

- Do you really have time to worry that one Rich Tea biscuit has four more calories than another? I don't think so.

- Is it helpful to tell you the calories per 100 g, leaving you to work out how much you are eating and how many calories it contains? Do you really want to carry a kitchen scales and a calculator when you're going to meet your friends in that hot new café? Life's too short!

With this handy little book you can forget all of those problems, because it gives you the real essentials, uniquely organised and calculated to make everything easy. It tells you how many calories you are consuming in everything you eat, from breakfast through to dinner – every snack and every drink, at home or eating out.

Most people who use this book will be doing so because they want to lose weight, but you can also use it if you want to gain weight. This at-a-glance calorie and nutrient ready-reckoner has all the information you need to achieve and maintain a healthy lifestyle, including great tips that really will make dieting easy.

A Healthy Lifestyle

Dieting of any kind, whether to lose or gain weight, should be part of a healthy lifestyle. Crank dieting is stupid and it doesn't work. If you try to lose weight by cutting out a particular food group, you may succeed, but you'll also become unfit and possibly even ill. In the same way, if you are trying to gain weight, eating mountains of sugary and fatty foods is not the answer.

Your body needs nutrients containing vitamins and minerals as well as the proper balance of protein, carbohydrate, fat and fibre to keep you fit and healthy. So as well as the calories, this book gives you the amounts of each of these food groups per portion of each food. With this information you can see which foods are good sources of which nutrient, and so ensure that you have the correct proportions each day.

Proteins

Your body needs protein to maintain good health and to repair itself when necessary. The best sources of proteins are fish, lean meat, poultry, dairy products, eggs and vegetable proteins such as pulses (dried peas, beans and lentils), tofu and Quorn. Eat two to three small portions of protein a day.

Carbohydrates

It may surprise you to know that complex carbohydrates, or starchy foods, should make up 50 per cent of each of your meals. This is because carbohydrates provide us with energy and are vital to our well-being. However, the added sugar (simple carbohydrates) and fat you mix with them will pile on the unwanted calories that can harm your health. The best sources are bread (all types), pasta, rice, cereals (this includes breakfast cereals but you should choose wholegrain varieties not sugar-coated ones) and potatoes. Eat plenty of all of these.

Vitamins and minerals

These are also essential for general good health. The best sources are fruit and vegetables. They should, preferably, be fresh, but frozen or canned in water or natural juice with no added sugar (and, ideally, no added salt) are fine. Eat at least five portions a day. See pages 12–15 for which foods are rich in which vitamins and minerals and why you need them.

Fat

You do need some fat in your diet – but not too much – to provide body warmth and energy. There is enough for your daily needs contained naturally in foods so keep added fat to a minimum and eat it sparingly (see my Clever diet tips for losing weight on pages 26–27).

Fibre

Your body also needs fibre – it is particularly necessary for your digestive function. Eat plenty of fruit and vegetables, wholegrain cereals, and the skins on potatoes.

Liquids

You also need lots of liquid in your diet. Make sure you drink plenty of water from the tap, filtered or mineral according to your preference. If you're really not keen on water, flavour it with a low-calorie squash.

Pure fruit juices are good for you and count as one portion of your five-a-day of fruit and vegetables however much you drink. The vitamin C in them helps you absorb the iron in foods such as fortified breakfast cereals too. Fruit drinks do contain calories, however, so they must be counted in your daily allowance.

Tea and coffee may be drunk in moderation but preferably after or between meals, as the tannin in the beverages impairs the absorption of some essential nutrients. If you want to add milk, use skimmed or semi-skimmed. Alternatively, drink both tea and coffee black (tea with lemon is deliciously refreshing and contains hardly any calories). Don't add any sugar. If you have a sweet tooth, use artificial sweeteners, but, ideally, wean yourself off them. Learning to do without sweetness will help your new, healthy lifestyle.

Try to consume at least 300 ml/½ pt/1¼ cups of skimmed or semi-skimmed milk during the day; this includes what you put on cereal or use in cooking. If you have a lot of weight to lose, then go for the skimmed option.

Alcohol

Alcohol is not a dieter's friend. If you are trying to lose weight, it piles on 'empty' calories, so have it as a treat only. Use low-calorie mixers with spirits and go for low-strength beers. If you like wine, try having a spritzer (wine diluted with sparkling water). Whatever you do, **don't** use drink as a substitute for good, nutritious food.

Regular exercise

An active body is more likely to be a healthy body. However, one mad burst of exercise a week at the gym isn't a good idea (although it's better than nothing). You need to take more frequent, regular exercise to reap the benefit.

There are plenty of ways to exercise without jogging or work-outs. Get into the habit of walking briskly instead of wandering along. Go on foot whenever possible instead of using the car or public transport. If you take the bus, get off a stop before your usual one and walk the last part of the journey. Ride a bike if you have one. Use the stairs instead of lifts or escalators. Take up a recreational sport like tennis or swimming or join an activity like a dance class. Even gardening will burn off calories.

Bending and stretching exercises will also help to tone your muscles but seek advice before you start any exercise regime – you must do them correctly or you can cause injury. If you are going to do exercises at home, do them at a fixed time, perhaps as soon as you get out of bed or before you have your shower or bath in the morning or evening. Try to make them a regular part of your daily routine, otherwise the novelty will wear off after a few days and you won't persevere.

Vitamin and minerals in foods

I mentioned earlier that a balanced diet of fresh foods should contain sufficient vitamins and minerals to keep your body healthy, and supplements should not be necessary for the vast majority of people. However, if you have been told that you are deficient in iron, for example, you may want to increase the number of iron-rich foods in your diet. You can consult the following tables to find the foods that are particularly rich in the major vitamins and minerals.

Vitamin	Important for	Vitamin-rich foods
Vitamin A	Colour and night vision; healthy skin and mucous membranes	Liver, fortified margarines, butter, eggs, whole milk products (e.g. full-fat cheeses), green, orange and red vegetables, fish liver oils
B Vitamin complex: Thiamin (B_1)	Conversion of carbohydrates to energy; function of the central nervous system	Bread and other cereals, milk and milk products, potatoes, meat, yeast extract
Riboflavin (B_2)	Conversion of carbohydrates, fats and proteins to energy; healthy skin and eyes	Fortified breakfast cereals, eggs, vegetables, milk and milk products, meat (especially offal), poultry, yeast extract
Niacin (Nicotinic acid)	Conversion of carbohydrates, fats and proteins to energy	Fortified breakfast cereals, bread, potatoes, meat and meat products, poultry, fish
Vitamin B_6	Conversion of proteins, fats and carbohydrates to energy; function of the central nervous system	Potatoes and other vegetables, pulses (dried peas, beans and lentils), fruit, meat and poultry, cereals
Vitamin B_{12}	Function of the central nervous system; production of red blood cells; growth	Meat and meat products (especially liver), cheese, milk, eggs, fish, yeast extract, fortified breakfast cereals
Folic acid	Function of the central nervous system; production of red blood cells	Wholegrain cereals, offal, green, leafy vegetables (especially raw ones), oranges

Vitamin	Important for	Vitamin-rich foods
Pantothenic acid	Conversion of fats and proteins to energy	Pulses, fortified cereals, offal, fresh vegetables, peanuts
Biotin	Conversion of fats and proteins to energy	Milk and milk products, fruit and vegetables, fish, egg yolk, cereals, offal
Vitamin C	Production of collagen for connective tissue, blood vessels and capillaries; support of the immune system and healing; absorption of iron; detoxification (for alcohol and drugs)	Potatoes, pure fruit juices, fruit, especially blackcurrants, strawberries, kiwis and citrus, vegetables, especially potatoes, green vegetables, (bell) peppers
Vitamin D	Growth and maintenance of healthy teeth and bones; absorption of calcium	Sunshine, butter, fortified margarines, fortified breakfast cereals, eggs, oily fish
Vitamin E	Protection of cell membranes; antioxidant	Wholegrain cereals, eggs, dark leafy vegetables, vegetable oils
Vitamin K	Metabolism of energy; blood clotting	Vegetables, especially brassicas (cabbage, cauliflower, etc.) and spinach
Essential fatty acids: Linoleic acid (Omega-3) Linolenic acid (Omega-6)	General good health	Oily fish, vegetable seeds and seed oils (including polyunsaturated margarines)

Mineral	Important for	Mineral-rich foods
Calcium	Healthy growth and development of bones and teeth; release of hormones in the body	Milk and milk products, canned fish (especially the bones), bread, green vegetables
Chromium	Activating insulin, which controls the use of glucose in the body	Most foods, particularly wholegrain cereals and vegetables
Copper	Production of enzymes, especially those involved with the blood and bones and the immune system; aiding neurotransmission; respiration of cells	Wholegrain cereals, vegetables, meat, oysters, nuts
Fluorine	Prevention of tooth decay	Fish, water, tea
Iodine	Regulation of many body processes, via the thyroid hormones	Meat, fish, eggs, milk and milk products, iodised salt
Iron	Formation of red blood cells; transportation and transfer of oxygen; metabolism of drugs	Potatoes and other vegetables, bread and cereal products, meat, especially offal
Magnesium	Muscle tone; enzyme activation, especially to break down proteins	Bread and cereal products, potatoes and other vegetables, milk, nuts

Mineral	Important for	Mineral-rich foods
Manganese	Maintenance of healthy cells; activation of enzymes; helping the utilisation of calcium and potassium	Nuts, wholegrain cereals, tea
Molybdenum	Production of many enzymes, especially for theformation of uric acid; and the metabolism of DNA	Most foods, particularly vegetables and pulses
Phosphorus	Production of all cells; aidingstorage of energy, membrane function, growth and reproduction	Bread and cereal products, meat and meat products, milk and milk products
Potassium	Maintenance of water levels in the body	Fruit and pure fruit juices, vegetables, milk, meat
Selenium	Production of an enzyme inred blood cells; protection of membranes	Fish, cheese, milk, eggs, meat (especially offal), cereals
Sodium and chlorine	Maintenance of water levels in the body	Bread and cereal products, meat products, milk, cooking and table salt
Zinc	Metabolism of bones; release of Vitamin A and insulin; activation of enzymes; growth; support of the immune system; taste	Milk and milk products, bread and cereal products, meat and meat products

Nutrition Labelling

There are two different food labelling systems in operation: the *What's Inside Guide* to GDAs (Guideline Daily Amounts) and the *Traffic Lights*.

The *What's Inside Guide* is the brainchild of the Food and Drink Association on behalf of the UK Food and Drink Manufacturing Industry. It tells you how many calories, and how much sugar, fat (including the amount of saturated fat) and salt are in your portion of food, plus the percentages of your daily average intake. You'll find it on some branded goods and it has been adopted by Tesco, Morrisons and Somerfield.

The *Traffic Lights* were introduced by the Food Standards Agency and tell you at a glance whether the product has a high (red), medium (amber) or low (green) amount of fat (including saturated fat), sugar and salt – the foods we should be cutting down on – and how many grams there are of each per serving. Asda, Sainsbury's, Waitrose, Co-op and M&S have chosen this system and other food manufacturers have opted for this too.

There are pros and cons for either system. Some say that many people don't understand percentages, so the *What's Inside Guide* is confusing. Others say that some healthy foods come out looking bad for you with the *Traffic Lights* when, in fact, they are excellent as part of a healthy diet. Take cheese, for instance. It will come up as red for fat because it does have a high fat content, but it is also rich in protein and calcium and, in small amounts, is an excellent food source. A product with lots of fruit in it would also come out as red because it has lots of natural sugar, yet fruit is good for you.

However your food is labelled, read it and the ingredients label and make an informed choice. Whichever system is being used, they are both a step in the right direction to helping consumers understand what products contain.

The recommended daily amounts of each food type for an average adult are:

	Male	**Female**
Calories	2500	2000
Fats	95g	70g
Of which saturated	30g	20g
Proteins	55g	45g
Carbohydrates	300g	230g
Of which sugars	120g	90g
Salt	6g	6g
Fibre	24g	24g

Controlling Your Weight

Calorie counting is an efficient way of controlling your diet and so adjusting your weight. To lose weight, your energy, or calorie, intake from food and drink (that's the calories in the food you eat) needs to be less than your energy output (the number of calories you burn up through activity). Strictly speaking, the measure we refer to as 'calories' should actually be called kilocalories (units of 1,000 calories) but they are always abbreviated to kcalories, or calories.

An avge man uses about 2,500 calories a day; a woman about 1,900 calories. The difference is partly because of size and partly because women tend to have a slower metabolic rate – they don't use up calories as quickly. The more active your lifestyle and the more exercise you undertake, the more calories you will use up.

If you only want to lose a small amount of weight and you want to do it fairly quickly, you should aim for a low daily calorie intake – say 1,500 calories for a man, 1,000 calories for a woman. But if you are planning a long-term, substantial weight reduction, it is much more effective to take it more slowly, aiming at, say, 1,900 calories per day for a man and 1,500 for a woman.

If you are underweight, of course, you will need to consume more calories than you burn in order to gain weight.

Your perfect weight

It is crucial that you are realistic about the weight you want to be. Having established the weight that you are aiming for, you should plan for a slow and steady weight loss, or gain, and work towards maintaining a healthy, balanced diet as your normal routine.

On page 21 is a chart, based on UK government statistics **(for adults only)**, which shows you how much you should weigh according to your height. Your bone structure will dictate whether you are at the lower end of the scale or higher up. The important thing is to be within the limits of ideal weight.

Weigh yourself first thing in the morning, preferably without clothes. If you weigh yourself when you are dressed, make sure you are wearing similar clothing each time. Check where you are on the table, then work out how much weight you need to lose or gain.

Once you've made that calculation and started your diet, weigh yourself on the same scales, in the same way, **once a week only.** Avoid the temptation to keep hopping on and off the scales, as weight fluctuates throughout the day and from day to day, which will only make you disheartened. There is usually a quick burst of weight loss in the first few days of a slimming diet, then the rate of loss will level off. Weighing yourself once a week will give you a much clearer picture of your progress. In the same way, if you are trying to put on weight, there may be an initial burst, then your weight will reach a plateau for a while before rising again.

Don't give up. If you are following a healthy and sensible balanced diet, you will be rewarded in the end.

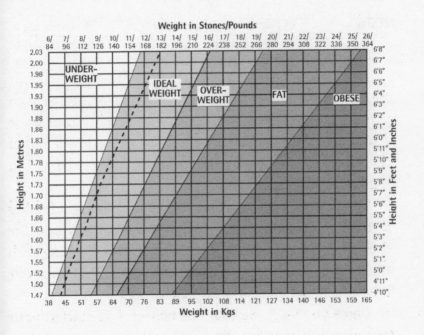

Calories and exercise

Regular exercise doesn't just burn up calories, it is a vital part of a healthy lifestyle. You'll see from this list (which is based on a woman of avge height and build) the difference between the number of calories you use up doing physically active tasks and the more leisurely ones.

Activity	Calories used in 30 minutes	Activity	Calories used in 30 minutes
Aerobics	210	House work	120
Ballroom dancing	190	Jogging	165
Climbing stairs	330	Manual work, heavy	225
Cycling, fast or uphill	330	Manual work, light	120
Cycling, leisurely speed	120	Running, fast	200
Disco dancing	205	Shopping	120
Driving a car	60	Sleeping	30
Gardening, digging	240	Squash	273
Gardening, hoeing	105	Swimming, racing speed	300
Golf	195	Swimming, relaxed speed	255
Gym work-out	210	Tennis	250
Hill-walking	240	Typing	60
Horse-riding, hacking	60	Walking, relaxed speed	120
Horse-riding, trotting and cantering	180	Walking, briskly	180
		Watching TV	45

Planning your diet

To keep a strict note of your calorie intake, you need to plan your day's menu, including drinks. Then look up each item and add the calorie totals together. The full amount should be equal to or less than your limit to lose weight; if you wish to gain weight, it should be above your limit. If the result is lower than your planned count for the day, you can give yourself an extra snack or another portion of healthy food, such as a vegetable or some bread with your meal. If you're over the limit and on a reducing diet, then you must find a lower-calorie alternative, perhaps grilled (broiled) fish instead of a fish pie, or fruit salad instead of apple crumble. To help you reduce your calorie count without even realising, I have included some cunning diet tips on pages 26–29.

Do read the tips for a healthy lifestyle on page 9, too. If you want your diet to work long-term and to keep fit and well, it is essential that you follow a sensible, balanced diet.

Going out for a meal

If you are trying to lose weight and you are invited out for a meal, don't panic. Most of the dishes you're likely to come across are in this book – even down to your aperitif or glass of wine. However, don't let yourself become a bore about it. Other people around you won't be dieting and if they see you constantly poring over your little guide, they will think you're obsessive. It's probably better to consult the book before you go out – you will soon get to know what are low-calorie foods and what are the blow-outs. Stick to the goodies if you can, but if you can't, don't worry. If you go over your calorie limit one day, then make sure the next day you stay under limit by a similar amount to even out your avge daily intake. But be warned, this will only work if you do it on an occasional basis. You can't expect to be able to cheat all the time. It's pointless to keep going over your limit, telling yourself that tomorrow you'll be good. Try to stick to your calorie limit every day, or you won't see the benefits.

Diet and health foods

There are many ranges of special diet foods available. They are relatively expensive, however, and do not offer any guarantee that you will actually lose weight. That said, low-calorie options can be useful when you are controlling your calories.

Regulations governing food labelling mean that the word 'diet' can appear on a label only if the food is a low-calorie one. In order to be so-named, it must contain no more than 40 calories per 100 g/4 oz or 100 ml/3½ fl oz and must state clearly that it can only help weight loss if consumed as part of a calorie-controlled diet.

Many foods claim to be nutritionally 'better for you' and there are voluntary guidelines in place over what some of these definitions mean. However, they can be rather vague, and some of the products that make this claim may be no better than the standard product. The only way to be sure is to read the labels (and this book!) and see the nutritional values for yourself. Below is a guide to what the wording on the labels means.

Fat-free	Contains no more than 0.15 g of fat per 100 g.
Low in saturates	Contains no more than 3 per cent saturated fat per 100 g.
Sugar-free	Contains no more than 0.2 g sugar per 100 g.
No added sugar	Has no sugar or foods made up mainly of sugars (e.g. dried fruit or concentrated fruit juice) added to it or any of its ingredients.
Reduced-fat/ reduced-sugar	Contains at least 25 per cent less fat/sugar than the standard product.
High fibre	Contains more than 6 g fibre per 100 g.
Low-fat/ low-sugar	Contains no more than 5 g fat/ sugar per 100 g.
Low-sodium	Contains no more than 40 mg sodium per 100 g.

All of the above are fairly clear. But there are other terms, commonly used on labels, that are not covered by the guidelines, and these can be more ambiguous.

Lower fat   This means the fat has less fat than the standard product, but the quantity may be reduced by only a tiny fraction!

Light or lite   This is likely to mean lower in fat but could mean lighter in weight, colour, or even texture! These, and lower fat foods, may have more sugar and starch (so more calories) to make them taste better.

Virtually fat-free   This should mean the food contains very little fat and so is a good one to look out for. But see below.

90 per cent fat-free   Sounds good – but in reality it means the product contains 10 per cent fat. This means it has more fat than one labelled 'low-fat'!

Clever diet tips for losing weight

You don't have to go on a special diet to lose weight – there are lots of ways to cut down on the calories whilst continuing to eat normal meals.

- Choose low-fat yoghurts, cheeses, cream, etc.
- Drink skimmed milk.
- Beware of cream substitutes – they often have more calories than the real thing!

- Fill up on as many vegetables or salad stuffs as you like – as long as they are not laced with gallons of oil or melted butter!
- Remove all fat or skin from meat and poultry before eating.
- Choose lean meats and trim off excess fat before cooking.
- Grill (broil) rather than fry (sauté).
- Use a low-fat spread instead of butter and add only a scraping to bread. Don't add any extra to vegetables before serving. I have given the calorie count for an avge spreading in the book. If you can use half that amount, do so (you will reap the benefits in reduced calories!)
- Beware of spread or butter melting into hot toast and 'clumping' on new bread – you won't be able to resist adding more!
- Use only the minimum of oil for cooking and drain off any excess.
- When browning meat for a made-up dish, dry-fry rather than adding oil and spoon off any fat.
- Don't add sugar to fruits, cereals or drinks.
- Choose low-calorie brands of soft drinks, dressings, etc.
- Drink plenty of water.
- Choose fruits canned in natural juice only, not syrup, and drink unsweetened pure juices. Beware of cartons labelled as fruit juice 'drinks' – these contain sugar and other additives.

Tips to make losing weight easier

Simply reducing the quantity of food you eat will help greatly in cutting down your calorie intake. If you are normally used to very large portions, try any of the following.

- Use a smaller plate for meals.
- A glass of naturally sparkling mineral water with your meal will help fill you up. Drink it in between meals too – zip it up with a slice of lemon or lime.
- Use a strong-flavoured cheese when cooking. You won't need to add so much to give it a good flavour.
- Cut foods into smaller pieces or thinner slices and serve yourself your usual number of pieces/slices – you'll think you've had the same but you'll actually have had less.
- Keep your butter or other spread at room temperature. It will spread much more easily, so you will use much less and save lots of calories. For example, a slice of bread and butter is 169 calories, but spread thinly with warm butter it will be only 132 calories!
- Chew slowly and eat small forkfuls. Your meal will last longer, giving you time to feel more satisfied.
- Never go shopping on an empty stomach – it's too tempting.
- Try to eat meals **before** you're ravenously hungry – especially if you are going to a restaurant!

- If you go out for a meal, don't skip the starter in the hope that you'll save calories. Opt for a low-calorie one – together with the main course it will take the edge off your appetite, and with any luck you'll be able to avoid the calorie-packed desserts!

- If you feel really peckish, eat some raw carrots – or any salad vegetables, or a bunch of grapes or a few slices of apple – to keep you going and take the edge off your appetite.

- Make a drink of meat or yeast extract (such as Bovril or Marmite) – a tsp in a mug of boiling water. It will take the edge off your appetite and help to fill you up between meals.

- Keep a packet of sugar-free chewing gum handy and chew between meals. Alternatively, clean your teeth instead of grabbing a snack – it really works!

- Always take the trouble to make your meal look appetising. A sprinkling of parsley or vegetables attractively arranged can help you really enjoy what's on your plate rather than just eating for the sake of it.

- Don't cheat! You know if you are piling food on your plate so try to be less-than-generous. Just remember, the smaller the portion, the more you'll lose. Avge portion means avge, not piled high!

- Don't weigh yourself more than once a week.

How to Use This Book

Using the book is simplicity itself. You will find everything from a slice of bread to a Tournedos rossini in here, and they are all easy to find.

- All the foods are listed alphabetically so that you can find them easily without having to work out a category or recall an obscure name.
- There are clear headings and dictionary-style page headings so you can easily flick through to the place you want to find.
- All the calories given are per portion, so you don't have anything to work out. It even gives you the avge calories for made-up dishes, so you don't have to weigh or calculate a thing.
- The amount of protein, carbohydrate and fat is listed for every item, plus a measure of the fibre content.
- If something may be found under two different names, I have included both and cross-referenced them.
- Prepared meals can be found under both the initial letter of the recipe title and also under the main ingredient. So Tandoori chicken may be found under both T for tandoori and C for chicken.

- Where a product has different variations, I have listed it under its generic name. So, for example, you'll find all the varieties of milk under M: 'Milk, skimmed', 'Milk, semi-skimmed' and so on.
- Where a food has different flavours, as do crisps (potato chips), for example, I have given an avge calorie content for all the flavours. You can always check the specific food labels for the exact calorie count, but the difference is only one or two calories!

Portion sizes

To make the book really dieter-friendly, I have calculated the foods using **average** portions (indicated as avge on the tables). To be sure of success with your diet, you must stick to these portion sizes. To make it clearer still – and harder for you to cheat – the table opposite explains exactly what I mean by each portion size. If you give yourself larger portions, you will suffer the consequences!

Food	Portion size given	Equivalent weight or size
Butter or other spreads	1 small knob	10 g/¼ oz/2 tsp
Cakes and pies	1 slice	⅛ of a standard pie or cake ⅙ large pizza or quiche
Cereals These vary according to type (flakes, porridge, etc.) and are based on manufacturer's recommended serving size. Use a large serving spoon, not a measuring spoon.	3 heaped tbsp 5 heaped tbsp	50 g or 40 g 40 g or 30 g
Cheese	1 small wedge/1 good spoonful/1 small chunk	25 g/1 oz
Chocolate	1 standard bar	One size up from fun size. (The standard bars vary but are on avge around 40 g.)
Drinks	1 small (beer/cider) 1 small glass	300 ml/½ pt/1¼ cups 100 ml/3½ fl oz/scant ½ cup
	1 wine glass 1 tumbler 1 mug 1 single measure 1 double measure	120 ml/4 fl oz/½ cup 200 ml/7 fl oz/scant 1 cup 250 ml/8 fl oz/1 cup 25 ml/1 fl oz/1½ tbsp 50 ml/2 fl oz/3 tbsp
Fish	1 (piece of) fillet/1 steak	175 g/6 oz
Fruit and vegetables	3 heaped tbsp 2 tbsp 1 good handful	100 g/4 oz 50 g/2 oz Approximately 25 g/1 oz (but it doesn't really matter as the calorie

content is tiny!)

Food	Portion size given	Equivalent weight or size
Ice cream	1 scoop	50 g/2 oz
Meat and poultry, roast	2 thick slices/3 med slices/4 thin slices	100 g/4 oz
Sandwiches	1 round	2 med slices of white bread, spread with butter, plus filling
Steaks	1 med steak	175 g/6 oz
	1 large steak (T-bone)	350 g/12 oz
Noodles, all types	1 serving	50 g/2 oz uncooked
Nuts and dried fruit	1 small handful	15 g/½ oz
Pasta, all types	1 serving	75 g/3 oz uncooked
Rice, all types and other grains	1 serving	50 g/2 oz/¼ cup uncooked
Soup	2 ladlefuls	200 ml/7 fl oz/scant 1 cup
	1 mug	250 ml/8 fl oz/1 cup
Sauces and sundries	1 tbsp	15 ml
	1 tsp	5 ml
Snacks	1 small bag	Crisps (chips): 25g Corn snacks, chocolate peanuts, etc: 50 g

Prepared dishes

For prepared dishes, whether home-made or bought ready-prepared, I have referred throughout to the measure '1 serving'. This means one standard, avge-sized serving. If the dish is home-made, and the recipe is designed to serve four people, '1 serving' denotes a quarter of the whole dish. In the same way, if a cook–chill or frozen meal is labelled as serving two, '1 serving' will be half the dish. If you eat the whole lot, you must double the calories!

Remember also that recipes vary, so you must be sensible about the content of those you choose. If you know the version you are cooking has loads of extra cream in it, don't kid yourself it is a standard one! When calculating the calorific and nutritional content of each item and recipe, I have estimated the content of an **average** portion and **average** recipe.

Brand names

The information has been gathered using both UK and American data. Obviously different brands of a product do not have identical nutritional values and manufacturers change their recipes from time to time, so the figures I have used are averages and may vary slightly from the brands you buy. Always read your labels for the latest and most precise data.

A–Z of Calorie Values

The easy-to-follow page headings and clear presentation mean that you will quickly and easily find the items you are looking for.

You can make your own notes on favourite brands, recipe ideas and healthy food combinations at the end of each section.

Food	kCal per portion	Portion size	Protein g	Carbs g	Fat g	Fibre
Abbey crunch biscuits (cookies)	**46**	1 biscuit	1	7	2	low
Absinthe	**55**	1 single measure	trace	trace	trace	0
Ace chocolate bar	**126**	1 standard bar	1	16	6	low
Aduki beans, dried, soaked and boiled	**123**	3 heaped tbsp	9	22	trace	high
Advocaat	**68**	1 single measure	1	7	2	0
Aero chocolate bar, mint	**254**	1 standard bar	3	28	13	0
Aero chocolate bar, orange	**254**	1 standard bar	3	28	13	0
Aero chocolate bar, milk	**251**	1 standard bar	3	26	13	0
Afelia (greek pork stew)	**369**	1 serving	24	12	28	low
After eight mints	**32**	1 mint	trace	6	1	0
Aioli	**237**	2 tbsp	trace	trace	23	0
Alfalfa sprouts	**7**	1 good handful	trace	1	trace	high
All-bran, dry	**68**	25 g/1 oz/½ cup	3	11	1	high
All-bran, with semi-skimmed milk	**139**	5 heaped tbsp	8	16	3	high
All-bran, with skimmed milk	**123**	5 heaped tbsp	8	16	1	high
Almond biscuits (cookies)	**46**	1 biscuit	1	6	2	low
Almond danish pastry	**420**	1 pastry	6	46	24	med
Almond macaroon	**120**	1 macaroon	3	13	7	med
Almond paste	**101**	25 g/1 oz	1	17	4	med
Almond slice	**132**	1 slice	2	21	5	low

Food	kCal per portion	Portion size	Protein g	Carbs g	Fat g	Fibre
Almonds, fresh, shelled	153	25 g/1 oz/¼ cup	5	2	14	high
Almonds, ground	46	1 tbsp	3	trace	4	high
Almonds, roasted	95	1 small handful	3	1	9	high
Almonds, sugared	15	1 sweet (candy)	trace	3	trace	high
Alpen, dry	91	25 g/1 oz/¼ cup	2	16	2	high
Alpen, with semi-skimmed milk	203	3 heaped tbsp	8	33	5	high
Alpen, with skimmed milk	189	3 heaped tbsp	8	33	3	high
Alpen, no added sugar, dry	89	25 g/1 oz/¼ cup	3	15	2	high
Alpen, no added sugar, with semi-skimmed milk	200	3 heaped tbsp	9	31	5	high
Alpen, no added sugar, with skimmed milk	184	3 heaped tbsp	9	31	3	high
Alpen nutty crunch, dry	95	25 g/1 oz/¼ cup	2	16	2	high
Alpen nutty crunch, with semi-skimmed milk	209	3 heaped tbsp	8	32	6	high
Alpen nutty crunch, with skimmed milk	193	3 heaped tbsp	8	32	4	high
Alphabetti spaghetti, canned	135	1 small can	4	28	1	med
Alphabetti spaghetti, on toast	304	1 small can plus 1 slice of buttered toast	7	46	9	med
Amaretti biscuits (cookies)	21	1 biscuit	trace	4	trace	low

Food	kCal per portion	Portion size	Protein g	Carbs g	Fat g	Fibre
Amaretto liqueur	80	1 single measure	0	7	0	0
American hard gums	135	1 small tube	2	40	0	0
American muffin, plain	169	1 muffin	5	24	6	med
American pancake	60	1 pancake	2	8	2	low
Anchovies, canned	12	1 fillet	1	0	1	0
Anchovies, fresh, grilled (broiled)	98	1 fish	15	0	4	0
Anchovy essence (extract)	7	1 tsp	1	0	trace	0
Anchovy paste	20	1 tbsp	3	trace	1	0
Angel cake	77	1 slice	1	12	trace	low
Angel delight, all flavours, made with semi-skimmed milk	115 (avge)	1 serving	3	16	4	0
Angel delight, all flavours, made with skimmed milk	105 (avge)	1 serving	3	16	2	0
Angel delight, sugar-free, all flavours, made with semi-skimmed milk	115 (avge)	1 serving	3	13	5	0
Angel delight, sugar-free, all flavours, made with skimmed milk	105 (avge)	1 serving	3	13	4	0
Angel hair (pasta, strands) dried, boiled	239	1 serving	8	51	2	med
Angel hair, fresh, boiled	301	1 serving	11	57	2	med
Angels on horseback	37	1 oyster plus ½ rasher (slice) of bacon	4	trace	3	0

Food	kCal per portion	Portion size	Protein g	Carbs g	Fat g	Fibre
Anis	55	1 single measure	trace	trace	0	0
Aniseed balls	81	1 small tube	trace	87	trace	0
Antipasti, mixed	244	1 serving	24	11	13	high
Anzac biscuits (cookies)	98	1 biscuit	2	4	5	low
Apple	47	1 fruit, unpeeled	trace	12	trace	high
Apple, cooking (tart)	35	1 large fruit, peeled	trace	9	trace	med
Apple, cooking, baked, sweetened	140	1 large fruit	1	12	trace	high
Apple, dried rings	13	1 ring	trace	3	trace	high
Apple, dried rings, stewed	66	3 heaped tbsp	trace	13	trace	high
Apple, dried rings, stewed with sugar	106	3 heaped tbsp	trace	17	trace	high
Apple, stewed	33	3 heaped tbsp	trace	8	trace	med
Apple, stewed with sugar	74	3 heaped tbsp	trace	19	trace	med
Apple, toffee	251	1 med fruit	4	66	trace	high
Apple amber	340	1 serving	2	14	2	med
Apple and blackcurrant juice drink	74	1 tumbler	trace	16	trace	0
Apple and mango juice drink	67	1 tumbler	0	13	trace	0
Apple betty	260	1 serving	2	39	10	med
Apple cake	252	1 slice	3	32	10	med
Apple charlotte	263	1 serving	3	41	9	med
Apple chutney	30	1 tbsp	trace	3	trace	low

Food	kCal per portion	Portion size	Protein g	Carbs g	Fat g	Fibre
Apple croissant	144	1 croissant	4	21	5	med
Apple crumble	297	1 serving	3	51	10	med
Apple danish pastry	298	1 pastry	6	51	18	med
Apple drink, sparkling	78	1 tumbler	trace	19	trace	0
Apple drink, sparkling, low-calorie	9	1 tumbler	trace	2	trace	0
Apple dumpling	287	1 dumpling	3	54	8	high
Apple fritter	136	1 fritter	2	26	5	med
Apple jelly (clear conserve)	67	1 tbsp	0	17	0	low
Apple juice, pure	76	1 tumbler	trace	10	trace	low
Apple juice drink, diluted	88	1 tumbler	trace	21	trace	0
Apple pie	290	1 slice	3	39	14	med
Apple sauce	25	1 tbsp	trace	2	trace	med
Apple snow	97	1 serving	4	19	1	med
Apple strudel	194	1 slice	2	29	8	med
Apple tango	78	1 tumbler	trace	19	trace	0
Apple tango, light	9	1 tumbler	trace	2	trace	0
Apple turnover	284	1 turnover	4	31	16	med
Apricot	17	1 fruit	trace	4	trace	med
Apricot and almond danish pastry	270	1 pastry	6	38	12	med
Apricot bites, dry	70	25 g/1 oz/½ cup	3	13	1	high
Apricot bites, with semi-skimmed milk	169	3 heaped tbsp	9	27	2	high

Food	kCal per portion	Portion size	Protein g	Carbs g	Fat g	Fibre
Apricot bites, with skimmed milk	153	3 heaped tbsp	9	27	3	high
Apricot brandy	56	1 single measure	trace	7	0	0
Apricot jam (conserve)	39	1 tbsp	trace	10	0	0
Apricot juice	78	1 tumbler	1	20	trace	0
Apricot nectar	112	1 tumbler	1	32	trace	0
Apricot sorbet	57	1 scoop	trace	19	trace	low
Apricots, canned in natural juice	34	3 heaped tbsp	trace	8	trace	med
Apricots, canned in syrup	63	3 heaped tbsp	trace	16	trace	med
Apricots, dried	15	1 fruit	trace	3	trace	high
Apricots, dried, stewed	85	3 heaped tbsp	1	22	trace	high
Apricots, dried, stewed with sugar	113	3 heaped tbsp	1	29	trace	high
Apricots, stewed	31	3 heaped tbsp	1	7	trace	med
Apricots, stewed with sugar	61	3 heaped tbsp	1	15	trace	med
Arbroath smokies, grilled (broiled), with butter	239	1 fish	37	0	10	0
Archers peach liqueur	65	1 single measure	trace	8	0	0
Arctic roll	100	1 slice	2	16	3	low
Arrowroot biscuits (cookies), thin	35	1 biscuit	1	7	2	low
Artichoke, globe, boiled	70	1 artichoke	0	3	0	med
Artichoke, with melted butter	181	1 artichoke	1	3	13	med

Food	kCal per portion	Portion size	Protein g	Carbs g	Fat g	Fibre
Artichoke hearts, canned, drained	8	1 heart	1	1	trace	med
Artichoke vinaigrette	211	1 artichoke	1	3	22	med
Artichokes, Jerusalem, boiled	41	3 heaped tbsp	2	11	0	high
Asparagus, canned, drained	24	½ med can	3	1	trace	med
Asparagus, roasted in olive oil	161	6 thick or 10 thin spears	3	1	16	med
Asparagus, steamed or boiled	26	6 thick or 10 thin spears	3	2	2	med
Asparagus, with melted butter	137	6 thick or 10 thin spears	3	1	13	med
Asparagus quiche	320	1 slice	13	18	22	med
Asparagus soup, cream of, canned	132	2 ladlefuls	2	10	10	low
Asparagus soup, cream of, instant	143	1 mug	1	20	6	low
Asparagus soup, home-made	167	2 ladlefuls	3	7	14	high
Aubergine (eggplant), fried (sautéed) in oil	302	¼ aubergine	1	3	32	med
Aubergine, steamed or boiled	28	¼ aubergine	1	3	trace	med
Aubergine, stuffed with meat	510	½ aubergine	46	28	24	med
Aubergine, stuffed with savoury rice	523	½ aubergine	8	26	14	high
Aubergine dip	20	2 tbsp	1	4	1	med

A

Food	kCal per portion	Portion size	Protein g	Carbs g	Fat g	Fibre
Austrian coffee cake	**488**	1 slice	5	41	32	low
Austrian smoked cheese	**60**	¼ barrel (25 g/1 oz)	4	trace	3	0
Avgolemono soup	**74**	2 ladlefuls	3	5	2	low
Avocado	**286**	1 med fruit	3	3	29	med
Avocado, baked, with tomato and cheese	**196**	½ avocado	5	4	18	med
Avocado, with prawns (shrimp) in cocktail sauce	**356**	½ avocado	13	2	32	med
Avocado vinaigrette	**240**	½ avocado	1	1	25	med

Food	kCal per portion	Portion size	Protein g	Carbs g	Fat g	Fibre
Babybel cheese	53	1 cheese	4	0	4	0
Bacardi	50	1 single measure	trace	trace	trace	0
Bacardi and coke	94	1 single measure plus 1 mixer	trace	6	0	0
Bacardi and diet coke	56	1 single measure plus 1 mixer	trace	trace	0	0
Baclava	322	1 pastry	5	40	17	med
Bacon, back, lean, fried (sautéed)	133	1 rasher (slice)	13	0	16	0
Bacon, back, lean, grilled (broiled)	117	1 rasher	12	0	8	0
Bacon, joint, boiled	325	2 thick slices	20	0	27	0
Bacon, joint, honey-roasted	346	2 thick slices	20	4	27	0
Bacon, streaky, fried	149	1 rasher	7	0	13	0
Bacon, streaky, grilled	127	1 rasher	7	0	11	0
Bacon and egg quiche	387	1 slice	15	17	31	low
Bacon and egg mcmuffin	346	1 muffin	20	26	18	med
Bacon and mushroom pizza, deep-pan	340	1 slice	10	35	16	med
Bacon and mushroom pizza, thin-crust	290	1 slice	10	25	15	med
Bacon cheeseburger	400	1 burger	24	27	22	low
Bacon sandwiches	538	1 round	30	34	32	med
Bagel	228	1 bagel	7	44	3	med
Bagna cauda	499	1 individual pot	6	0	52	0

Food	kCal per portion	Portion size	Protein g	Carbs g	Fat g	Fibre
Baguette	**364**	1 small	11	75	2	med
Bailey's irish cream	**80**	1 single measure	trace	6	4	0
Baked alaska	**339**	1 serving	8	62	8	low
Baked beans	**168**	1 small can	10	31	1	high
Baked beans, barbecued	**164**	1 small can	10	30	1	high
Baked beans, on toast	**323**	1 small can plus 1 slice of toast	14	49	10	high
Baked beans, reduced-sugar and reduced-salt	**146**	1 small can	11	25	1	high
Baked beans, reduced-sugar and reduced-salt, on toast	**301**	1 small can plus 1 slice of toast	14	43	10	high
Baked beans, with bacon	**182**	1 small can plus 2 rashers (slices) of bacon	12	26	3	high
Baked beans, with burgers, canned	**206**	1 small can	13	26	6	high
Baked beans, with sausages, canned	**220**	1 small can	10	26	9	high
Baked beans, with vegetarian sausages, canned	**240**	1 small can	11	63	trace	high
Bakewell slice	**156**	1 slice	1	22	7	med
Bakewell tart	**297**	1 slice	4	37	15	med
Balsamic condiment	**1**	1 tsp	trace	1	0	0
Bamboo shoots	**6**	2 tbsp	1	trace	trace	med

Food	kCal per portion	Portion size	Protein g	Carbs g	Fat g	Fibre
Banana	95	1 medium fruit	1	23	trace	med
Banana, dried slices	78	1 small handful	trace	9	5	med
Banana bread	246	1 slice	2	45	7	med
Banana custard	50	5 tbsp	1	8	1	0
Banana flambé	250	1 banana	1	28	8	med
Banana fritter	175	1 fritter	3	33	5	med
Banana milkshake, fresh, made with semi-skimmed milk	163	1 tumbler	6	31	3	med
Banana milkshake, fresh, made with skimmed milk	144	1 tumbler	6	31	trace	med
Banana sandwiches	399	1 round	7	57	17	med
Banana split	481	1 serving	10	77	16	med
Bananabix, dry	92	25 g/1 oz/½ cup	2	18	trace	high
Bananabix, with semi-skimmed milk	207	3 heaped tbsp	8	35	4	high
Bananabix, with skimmed milk	191	3 heaped tbsp	8	35	3	high
Bangers and mash	462	2 sausages plus 4 spoonfuls of mash	17	43	20	med
Banoffee pie	574	1 slice	10	68	23	med
Barbecue sauce	11	1 tbsp	trace	1	trace	0
Barbecued baked beans	164	1 small can	10	30	1	high
Barbecued chicken	287	1 chicken portion	46	1	10	0
Barbecued pork chop	210	1 chop	28	1	9	0

Food	kCal per portion	Portion size	Protein g	Carbs g	Fat g	Fibre
Barbecued spare ribs	288	2 ribs	25	2	16	0
Barley sugar	96	1 stick	trace	24	0	0
Barley water, all flavours	40 (avge)	1 tumbler	trace	9	trace	0
Barley water, all flavours, no added sugar	6 (avge)	1 tumbler	trace	1	trace	0
Barley wine	120	1 small bottle	1	11	trace	0
Bass, fried (sautéed), in seasoned flour	261	1 piece of fillet	32	5	12	low
Bass, grilled (broiled)	142	1 piece of fillet	31	0	2	0
Bass, poached	141	1 piece of fillet	32	0	2	0
Bass, stuffed, baked	182	1 serving	32	1	4	low
Bath bun	263	1 bun	8	45	15	med
Bath olivers	50	1 biscuit (cookie)	1	8	2	low
Battenburg cake	370	1 slice	6	50	17	med
Bavarian smoked cheese	60	¼ barrel (25 g/1 oz)	4	trace	3	0
Bavarois, all flavours	308 (avge)	1 serving	7	17	23	0
Bean and cheese enchiladas	547	2 enchiladas	28	82	14	high
Bean salad	120	3 heaped tbsp	4	12	5	high
Beanburger, spicy	112	1 burger	9	4	6	med
Beans See individual varieties, e.g. Runner beans						

Food	kCal per portion	Portion size	Protein g	Carbs g	Fat g	Fibre
Beansprouts	8	1 good handful	1	1	trace	high
Béarnaise sauce	275	5 tbsp	3	7	27	low
Béchamel sauce, made with semi-skimmed milk	96	5 tbsp	3	8	6	low
Beef, boiled	326	2 thick slices	28	0	24	0
Beef, corned	54	1 slice	7	0	3	0
Beef, grillsteak, grilled (broiled)	185	1 steak	11	8	12	low
Beef, minced (ground), in gravy, canned	230	½ large can	19	14	11	0
Beef, minced, lean, stewed	229	1 serving	23	0	15	0
Beef, roast, lean	225	4 thin slices	28	0	19	0
Beef, steak *See* Steak						
Beef, stewed in gravy	335	1 serving	47	0	16	0
Beef, stewed in gravy, canned	254	½ large can	32	8	10	0
Beef and cheese enchiladas	644	2 enchiladas	24	60	36	low
Beef and tomato soup, canned	88	2 ladlefuls	5	10	2	low
Beef and tomato soup, instant	72	1 mug	1	15	1	0
Beef and vegetable stir-fry	433	1 serving	26	71	5	high
Beef broth, canned	76	2 ladlefuls	4	13	1	low

Food	kCal per portion	Portion size	Protein g	Carbs g	Fat g	Fibre
Beef carbonnade (in beer)	**384**	1 serving	30	15	21	low
Beef casserole	**360**	1 serving	28	13	21	med
Beef chop suey	**297**	1 serving	23	34	6	med
Beef chow mein	**408**	1 serving	19	43	18	high
Beef consommé, canned	**14**	2 ladlefuls	3	1	trace	0
Beef consommé, jellied	**21**	2 ladlefuls	4	1	trace	0
Beef curry, home-made	**905**	1 serving	37	10	77	med
Beef curry, home-made, with rice	**1153**	1 serving	42	66	79	med
Beef curry, retail	**411**	1 serving	40	19	18	med
Beef curry, retail, with rice	**657**	1 serving	43	82	19	med
Beef fajitas	**528**	2 fajitas	40	79	8	med
Beef goulash	**406**	1 serving	28	16	22	med
Beef in oyster sauce	**204**	1 serving	24	10	8	low
Beef kheema	**826**	1 serving	36	1	75	low
Beef koftas	**441**	1 serving	28	4	35	low
Beef olives	**494**	2 olives	58	20	18	low
Beef pie	**460**	1 individual pie	18	32	28	low
Beef pot roast, with vegetables	**420**	1 serving	44	14	15	med
Beef risotto	**452**	1 serving	16	54	29	low
Beef satay	**222**	1 skewer	25	6	11	low

Food	kCal per portion	Portion size	Protein g	Carbs g	Fat g	Fibre
Beef sausages, thick, fried (sautéed)	**108**	1 sausage	5	6	7	low
Beef sausages, thick, grilled (broiled)	**106**	1 sausage	5	6	7	low
Beef sausages, thin, fried	**54**	1 sausage	3	4	4	low
Beef sausages, thin, grilled	**53**	1 sausage	3	4	4	low
Beef spread	**35**	1 tbsp	1	2	3	low
Beef steak pudding	**684**	1 serving	33	57	37	med
Beef stew	**360**	1 serving	28	13	21	med
Beef stroganoff	**361**	1 serving	22	8	25	med
Beef teriyaki	**128**	1 serving	18	2	4	low
Beef wellington	**527**	1 serving	37	23	33	low
Beef with mushrooms, chinese	**320**	1 serving	37	44	6	low
Beef with pineapple, chinese	**337**	1 serving	23	47	6	low
See also Boeuf						
Beefburger, fried (sautéed)	**125**	1 burger	6	trace	11	0
Beefburger, grilled (broiled)	**122**	1 burger	6	trace	11	0
Beefburger, in a bun, quarterpounder	**321**	1 burger in a bun	22	27	15	med
Beefburger, in a bun, small	**246**	1 burger in a bun	11	23	13	med

Food	kCal per portion	Portion size	Protein g	Carbs g	Fat g	Fibre
Beer, bitter	96	1 small	1	7	trace	0
Beer, extra-strength	216	1 small	2	18	trace	0
Beer, pale ale	96	1 small	1	6	trace	0
Beerwurst	55	1 slice	3	trace	4	0
Beetroot (red beet)	36	1 med	2	7	trace	med
Beetroot, boiled	46	1 med	2	9	trace	med
Beetroot, pickled	28	5 slices	1	6	trace	med
Bel paese cheese	87	1 small wedge	5	trace	7	0
Belgian bun	192	1 bun	5	30	5	low
Belgian endive See Chicory						
Belgian ham, dry-cured	21	1 slice	4	0	1	0
Bell pepper See Pepper						
Benedictine	90	1 single measure	0	6	0	0
Big bar ace	204	1 standard bar	2	25	10	low
Big breakfast	591	1 meal	26	40	36	high
Big fish sandwich	720	1 bun	23	59	43	high
Big mac	493	1 burger	27	44	23	high
Bigarde sauce	123	5 tbsp	5	10	4	low
Biscotti	39	1 biscuit (cookie)	1	6	1	low
Biscuits (cookies), chocolate, full-coated	131	1 biscuit	1	17	7	low
Biscuits, chocolate, half-coated	84	1 biscuit	1	11	4	low
Biscuits, cream-filled	77	1 biscuit	1	10	4	low

Food	kCal per portion	Portion size	Protein g	Carbs g	Fat g	Fibre
Biscuits, semi-sweet	46	1 biscuit	1	7	2	low
Biscuits, short, sweet	47	1 biscuit	1	6	2	low
Biscuits, wafer, cream-filled	39	1 biscuit	trace	5	3	low
See also individual names, e.g. Hobnob						
Bitter lemon, sparkling	68	1 tumbler	trace	16	0	0
Bitter orange, sparkling	68	1 tumbler	trace	16	0	0
Black bean sauce	22	1 tbsp	1	3	trace	low
Black beans, dried, soaked and cooked	103	3 heaped tbsp	trace	18	trace	high
Black cherries, canned in syrup	71	3 heaped tbsp	0	18	trace	low
Black cherry cheesecake	242	1 slice	6	33	11	low
Black cherry jam (conserve)	39	1 tbsp	trace	10	0	0
Black cherry jam, reduced-sugar	6	1 tbsp	trace	5	0	0
Black forest gateau	432	1 slice	7	65	18	low
Black forest ham	29	1 thin slice	4	trace	2	0
Black gram, boiled	45	1 serving	4	7	trace	low
Black jack chew sweets (candies)	15	1 sweet	0	3	trace	0
Black pudding, fried (sautéed)	305	2 thick slices	13	15	22	low
Black velvet	168	1 cocktail	1	5	0	0

Food	kCal per portion	Portion size	Protein g	Carbs g	Fat g	Fibre
Blackberries	25	3 heaped tbsp	1	5	trace	high
Blackberries, stewed	21	3 heaped tbsp	1	4	trace	med
Blackberries, stewed with sugar	56	3 heaped tbsp	1	14	trace	med
Blackberry and apple crumble	297	1 serving	3	51	10	med
Blackberry and apple pie	281	1 slice	3	11	39	med
Blackberry jam (conserve)	39	1 tbsp	trace	10	0	0
Blackcurrant and apple pie	378	1 slice	3	56	16	med
Blackcurrant and apple squash, diluted	58	1 tumbler	0	15	0	0
Blackcurrant cheesecake	260	1 slice	3	38	12	low
Blackcurrant cordial, diluted	103	1 tumbler	trace	27	0	0
Blackcurrant crumble	298	1 serving	3	51	10	med
Blackcurrant jam (conserve)	39	1 tbsp	trace	10	0	0
Blackcurrant jam, reduced-sugar	6	1 tbsp	trace	5	0	0
Blackcurrant juice drink	120	1 tumbler	trace	32	trace	0
Blackcurrant pastilles	131	1 small tube	3	32	0	0
Blackcurrant pie	282	1 slice	3	34	13	med
Blackcurrant sorbet	65	1 scoop	trace	17	trace	0
Blackcurrants	28	3 heaped tbsp	1	7	trace	high

Food	kCal per portion	Portion size	Protein g	Carbs g	Fat g	Fibre
Blackcurrants, canned in natural juice	31	3 heaped tbsp	1	8	trace	med
Blackcurrants, canned in syrup	72	3 heaped tbsp	1	18	trace	med
Blackcurrants, stewed with sugar	58	3 heaped tbsp	1	15	trace	med
Black-eyed beans, dried, soaked and cooked	116	3 heaped tbsp	9	20	1	high
Blancmange	165	1 serving	5	23	6	low
Blewits, fried (sautéed)	78	2 tbsp	1	trace	8	low
Blewits, stewed	6	2 tbsp	1	trace	trace	low
Blinis	60	1 pancake	2	8	2	low
Blintzes	86	1 pancake	8	11	1	low
Bloater, grilled (broiled)	298	1 fish	31	0	19	0
Bloater paste	5	1 tsp	trace	1	trace	low
Bloody mary	69	1 cocktail	1	3	trace	low
Bloomer loaf	70	1 med slice	3	15	1	low
BLT	650	1 round	30	34	35	med
Blue brie cheese	106	1 small wedge	4	trace	10	0
Blue chartreuse	78	1 single measure	trace	7	0	0
Blue cheese dip	145	1 small pot	1	trace	12	0
Blue cheese dressing	77	1 tbsp	1	1	8	0
Blue cheese dressing, low-calorie	16	1 tbsp	trace	2	1	0
Blue riband chocolate wafer	108	1 standard bar	1	13	6	low

Food	kCal per portion	Portion size	Protein g	Carbs g	Fat g	Fibre
Blue stilton cheese	103	1 small wedge	6	trace	9	0
Blueberries	56	3 heaped tbsp	1	14	trace	med
Blueberries, canned in syrup	88	3 heaped tbsp	1	22	trace	med
Blueberries, dried	44	1 small handful	trace	12	trace	high
Blueberries, stewed	51	3 heaped tbsp	trace	12	trace	med
Blueberries, stewed with sugar	81	3 heaped tbsp	trace	22	trace	med
Blueberry buster muffin	408	1 muffin	4	47	21	med
Blueberry muffin	294	1 large muffin	5	38	14	med
Blueberry pie	290	1 slice	3	39	14	med
Bluefish, grilled (broiled)	186	1 fillet	30	0	6	0
Boasters biscuits (cookies), all flavours	90 (avge)	1 biscuit	1	20	5	low
Bockwurst	199	1 sausage	9	trace	18	0
Boeuf bourguignon	450	1 serving	31	7	33	low
Boeuf en daube	351	1 serving	39	14	13	med
See also Beef						
Boiled beef with carrots and dumplings	474	1 serving	36	29	26	med
Boiled sweets (candies)	15	1 sweet	trace	5	trace	0
Bologna sausage	57	1 slice	3	trace	5	0
Bolognese sauce	217	1 serving	12	5	17	low
Bolony sausage	57	1 slice	3	trace	5	0
Bombay mix snack	75	1 small handful	1	2	5	high

Food	kCal per portion	Portion size	Protein g	Carbs g	Fat g	Fibre
Bon bel cheese	78	1 small wedge	6	0	6	0
Bon-bons	28	1 sweet (candy)	0	6	trace	0
Bonito, grilled (broiled)	195	1 piece of fillet	34	0	7	0
Boost chocolate bar	295	1 standard bar	3	34	16	low
Bordelaise sauce	133	5 tbsp	5	2	4	0
Borlotti beans, canned, drained	112	3 heaped tbsp	5	8	trace	high
Borlotti beans, dried, soaked and cooked	116	3 heaped tbsp	6	18	1	high
Bortsch	25	2 ladlefuls	3	1	1	high
Bortsch, jellied	50	2 ladlefuls	9	1	1	high
Boston baked beans	133	1 serving	7	26	1	high
Boudoir biscuits (lady fingers)	40	1 finger	1	6	1	low
Bouillabaisse	159	2 ladlefuls	16	21	2	med
Bouillabaise with rouille	310	2 ladlefuls	17	23	17	med
Bounty bar, milk chocolate	289	1 standard bar	3	32	15	low
Bounty bar, plain (semi-sweet) chocolate	276	1 standard bar	2	33	15	low
Bounty, ice cream bar	299	1 standard bar	4	24	21	low
Bourbon	60	1 single measure	trace	trace	0	0
Bourbon biscuits (cookies)	63	1 biscuit	1	9	3	low
Bournville chocolate	250	1 standard bar	2	30	13	0
Bournvita, made with semi-skimmed milk	145	1 mug	9	19	4	low

Food	kCal per portion	Portion size	Protein g	Carbs g	Fat g	Fibre
Bournvita, made with skimmed milk	**137**	1 mug	9	20	2	low
Boursin cheese,	**77** (avge)	1 heaped tbsp	2	1	7	0
Boursin, light, all flavours	**28** (avge)	1 heaped tbsp	2	1	2	0
Bovril	**3**	1 tsp	2	trace	trace	0
Bran, oat	**51**	1 tbsp	2	9	1	high
Bran, wheat	**31**	1 tbsp	2	4	1	high
Bran muffin	**163**	1 muffin	4	24	6	high
Brandy	**55**	1 single measure	trace	trace	0	0
Brandy alexander	**270**	1 cocktail	trace	6	18	0
Brandy butter	**73**	1 tbsp	trace	8	4	0
Brandy sauce, made with semi-skimmed milk	**50**	5 tbsp	1	5	2	low
Brandy sauce, made with skimmed milk	**47**	5 tbsp	1	5	trace	low
Brandy snaps	**57**	1 snap	trace	10	2	low
Brandy sour	**57**	1 cocktail	trace	trace	trace	0
Branflakes, dry	**80**	25 g/1 oz/½ cup	2	16	1	high
Branflakes, with semi-skimmed milk	**185**	5 heaped tbsp	8	33	3	high
Branflakes, with skimmed milk	**169**	5 heaped tbsp	8	33	1	high
Branflakes, with sultanas (golden raisins), dry	**80**	25 g/1 oz/½ cup	2	16	trace	high

Food	kCal per portion	Portion size	Protein g	Carbs g	Fat g	Fibre
Branflakes, with sultanas, with skimmed milk	**169**	5 heaped tbsp	8	33	1	high
Branflakes, with sultanas, with semi-skimmed milk	**185**	5 heaped tbsp	8	33	3	high
Bratwurst, fried (sautéed)	**256**	1 sausage	12	2	22	0
Brazil nut, shelled	**23**	1 nut	1	trace	3	high
Brazil nut toffee	**39**	1 toffee	trace	5	2	low
Brazils, chocolate	**49**	1 sweet (candy)	1	3	4	high
Bread, brown, med-sliced	**78**	1 slice	3	16	1	med
Bread, brown, med-sliced, toasted	**80**	1 slice	3	16	1	med
Bread, brown, thick-sliced	**109**	1 slice	4	22	1	med
Bread, brown, thin-sliced	**65**	1 slice	2	13	1	med
Bread, granary, med-sliced	**94**	1 slice	4	18	1	med
Bread, granary, med-sliced, toasted	**96**	1 slice	4	18	1	med
Bread, granary, thick-sliced	**117**	1 slice	5	23	2	med
Bread, softgrain med-sliced,	**76**	1 slice	3	15	1	med
Bread, softgrain, med-sliced, toasted	**85**	1 slice	3	18	1	med

Food	kCal per portion	Portion size	Protein g	Carbs g	Fat g	Fibre
Bread, softgrain, thick-sliced	**106**	1 slice	5	21	1	med
Bread, white, med-sliced	**78**	1 slice	3	17	trace	low
Bread, white, med-sliced, toasted	**81**	1 slice	3	18	trace	low
Bread, white, thick-sliced	**108**	1 slice	4	23	trace	low
Bread, white, thin-sliced	**65**	1 slice	2	14	trace	low
Bread, wholemeal, med-sliced	**77**	1 slice	3	15	1	high
Bread, wholemeal, med-sliced, toasted	**79**	1 slice	3	15	1	high
Bread, wholemeal, thick-sliced	**107**	1 slice	5	21	1	high
Bread, wholemeal, thin-sliced	**64**	1 slice	3	12	1	high
Bread, with butter	**152** (avge)	1 med slice	3	17	9	low
Bread, with low-fat spread	**117** (avge)	1 med slice	3	17	4	low
Bread pudding	**297**	1 serving	6	50	10	med
Bread and butter pudding	**280**	1 serving	10	31	13	low
Bread roll, baton	**182**	1 roll	6	38	1	med
Bread roll, brown	**134**	1 roll	5	26	2	med
Bread roll, crusty	**140**	1 roll	5	29	2	low
Bread roll, finger	**107**	1 roll	4	21	2	low
Bread roll, granary	**117**	1 roll	5	23	1	med

Food	kCal per portion	Portion size	Protein g	Carbs g	Fat g	Fibre
Bread roll, hamburger bun	**132**	1 bun	4	24	2	low
Bread roll, soft white bap	**134**	1 roll	5	26	2	low
Bread roll, starch-reduced	**50**	1 roll	2	10	trace	low
Bread roll, wholemeal	**120**	1 roll	4	24	1	high
Bread roll, with butter	**214** (avge)	1 roll	13	29	9	low
Bread roll, with low-fat spread	**179** (avge)	1 roll	14	29	5	low
Bread sauce, made with semi-skimmed milk	**14**	1 tbsp	1	2	trace	low
Bread sauce, made with skimmed milk	**12**	1 tbsp	1	2	trace	low
Breadfruit	**396**	1 med fruit	4	104	trace	high
Breadfruit, canned, drained	**66**	3 heaped tbsp	1	16	trace	med
Breadsticks	**20**	1 stick	1	3	trace	low
Breakaway chocolate bar, caramac	**125**	1 standard bar	1	13	7	low
Breakaway, milk	**114**	1 standard bar	1	14	6	low
Breakfast compôte, canned	**73**	3 heaped tbsp	trace	17	trace	high
Bream, fried (sautéed) in seasoned flour	**261**	1 piece of fillet	32	5	12	low
Bream, grilled (broiled)	**142**	1 piece of fillet	31	0	2	0
Bream, poached	**141**	1 piece of fillet	32	0	2	0
Bresaola	**15**	1 thin slice	3	trace	trace	0

Food	kCal per portion	Portion size	Protein g	Carbs g	Fat g	Fibre
Bresse bleu cheese	106	1 small wedge	4	trace	10	0
Brie cheese	80	1 small wedge	5	trace	7	0
Brill, fried (sautéed) in egg and breadcrumbs	342	1 piece of fillet	27	13	20	low
Brill, grilled (broiled)	126	1 piece of fillet	23	0	3	0
Brill, poached	125	1 piece of fillet	25	0	2	0
Brioche	140	1 brioche	4	22	4	low
Brisket of beef, boiled	326	2 thick slices	28	0	24	0
Broad (fava) beans, boiled	48	3 heaped tbsp	5	6	1	high
Broad beans, canned, drained	77	3 heaped tbsp	6	13	trace	high
Broad beans, frozen, cooked	81	3 heaped tbsp	8	12	1	high
Broccoli, steamed or boiled	33	4 med florets	4	2	1	med
Broccoli and cauliflower soup, instant	59	1 mug	1	8	2	low
Broccoli and cauliflower soup, packet	110	2 ladlefuls	2	15	5	med
Broccoli and cheese quiche	320	1 slice	13	18	22	low
Broccoli and cheese soup, canned	132	2 ladlefuls	4	9	7	med
Broccoli and cheese soup, home-made	169	2 ladlefuls	9	21	6	high
Broccoli in cheese sauce, made with semi-skimmed milk	167	1 serving	10	9	11	med

Food	kCal per portion	Portion size	Protein g	Carbs g	Fat g	Fibre
Broccoli in cheese sauce, made with skimmed milk	157	1 serving	10	9	11	med
Broccoli soup	118	2 ladlefuls	6	21	2	high
Brown ale	84	1 small	1	9	trace	0
Brown betty	260	1 serving	2	39	10	med
Brown sauce	15	1 tbsp	trace	4	0	low
Brownie, chocolate	368	1 brownie	5	63	11	med
Brunswick stew	444	1 serving	39	46	12	high
Brussels sprouts, steamed or boiled	35	3 heaped tbsp	3	3	1	high
Brussels sprouts, with chestnuts	176	3 heaped tbsp	2	20	43	high
Bubble and squeak	240	1 serving	3	7	18	high
Bucatini (long macaroni), dried, boiled	239	1 serving	8	51	2	med
Bucatini, fresh, boiled	301	1 serving	11	57	2	med
Buck rarebit	312	1 slice	17	22	19	low
Buckling, smoked	520	1 fish	26	0	44	0
Buckwheat noodles, boiled	228	1 serving	11	48	trace	low
Buckwheat pancakes	45	1 pancake	2	6	2	low
Bulgar (cracked wheat), cooked	177	3 heaped tbsp	6	29	4	med
Buns See individual flavours, e.g. Currant bun						

Food	kCal per portion	Portion size	Protein g	Carbs g	Fat g	Fibre
Burger bun	132	1 bun	4	24	2	low
Burgers See individual varieties, e.g. Hamburger						
Burritos, with beans and cheese	377	2 burritos	15	55	12	med
Burritos, with beef, beans and cheese	331	2 burritos	15	40	13	med
Butter	184	25 g/1 oz/2 tbsp	trace	trace	20	0
Butter	74	1 small knob	trace	trace	8	0
Butter (lima) beans, canned, drained	77	3 heaped tbsp	6	13	trace	high
Butter beans, dried, soaked and cooked	103	3 heaped tbsp	7	18	1	high
Butter pecan ice cream	91	1 scoop	2	12	4	low
Butter puffs	54	1 biscuit	1	6	3	low
Butter sauce	112	5 tbsp	3	8	8	low
Butter shortcake biscuits (cookies)	50	1 biscuit	1	7	2	low
Butter/vegetable fat spread	165	25 g/1 oz/2 tbsp	trace	trace	18	0
Butter/vegetable fat spread	66	1 small knob	trace	trace	7	0
Buttercream icing (frosting)	40	1 tbsp	trace	9	3	0
Butterfly cakes	245	1 individual cake	2	26	15	low
Butterfly prawns (jumbo shrimp), fried (sautéed), in breadcrumbs	405	6 prawns	16	35	23	low

Food	kCal per portion	Portion size	Protein g	Carbs g	Fat g	Fibre
Buttermilk	60	150 ml/¼ pt/ ⅔ cup	6	8	trace	0
Butternut squash, steamed or boiled	9	½ medium squash	trace	2	trace	low
Butterscotch	24	1 piece	trace	5	trace	0
Butterscotch sauce	145	2 tbsp	1	32	2	low
Butterscotch tart	531	1 slice	10	57	23	low

Food	kCal per portion	Portion size	Protein g	Carbs g	Fat g	Fibre
Cabbage, green, steamed or boiled	**16**	3 heaped tbsp	1	2	trace	med
Cabbage, red/white, pickled	**3**	1 tbsp	trace	trace	0	med
Cabbage, red/white, raw	**27**	3 heaped tbsp	1	5	trace	med
Cabbage leaves, stuffed	**221**	2 leaves	18	19	9	high
Cabinet pudding	**233**	1 serving	3	36	2	med
Caerphilly cheese	**94**	1 small wedge	6	trace	8	0
Caesar salad	**207**	1 serving	17	6	13	med
Café noir biscuits (cookies)	**39**	1 biscuit	trace	8	trace	low
Caffé latte	**133**	1 med cup	6	10	8	0
Cajun chicken	**366**	1 serving	40	33	9	0
Cake, chocolate	**384**	1 slice	5	58	14	low
Cake, light fruit	**354**	1 slice	5	58	13	med
Cake, plain	**393**	1 slice	5	58	17	low
Cake, rich fruit	**341**	1 slice	4	60	11	med
See also Sponge cake *and individual flavours, e.g.* Coffee cake						
Calabrese, steamed or boiled	**33**	4 medium florets	4	2	1	med
Calamari rings, fried (sautéed), in batter	**235**	1 serving	14	19	12	low
Calippo ice lolly, any flavour	**105**	1 lolly	trace	26	trace	0
Calvados	**55**	1 single measure	trace	trace	0	0

Food	kCal per portion	Portion size	Protein g	Carbs g	Fat g	Fibre
Calves' liver, braised	165	3 thin slices	22	3	7	low
Calves' liver, fried (sautéed), in seasoned flour	254	3 thin slices	27	7	13	0
Calypso coffee	218	1 wine glass	1	7	14	0
Calzone	470	1 individual pie	18	50	24	med
Cambozola cheese	106	1 small wedge	4	trace	10	0
Camembert cheese	74	1 small wedge	5	trace	6	0
Camp coffee, made with semi-skimmed milk	125	1 mug	8	15	4	0
Camp coffee, made with skimmed milk	93	1 mug	8	15	trace	0
Candied fruits *See* Glacé fruits						
Candied peel *See* Mixed peel						
Candy *See individual varieties, e.g.* Chocolate brazils, Lemon drops						
Candy floss	100	1 stick	trace	26	0	0
Cannellini beans, canned, drained	101	3 heaped tbsp	8	22	1	high
Cannellini beans, dried, soaked and cooked	103	3 heaped tbsp	8	17	trace	high
Cannelloni, filled with meat	298	2 tubes	12	24	17	med
Cannelloni, filled with spinach and ricotta	250	2 tubes	9	17	16	med
Cantal cheese	101	1 small wedge	6	trace	8	0

Food	kCal per portion	Portion size	Protein g	Carbs g	Fat g	Fibre
Canteloupe melon	57	½ melon	2	13	trace	med
Cape gooseberries	3	1 fruit	trace	trace	trace	low
Cappellini (pasta strands), dried, boiled	239	1 serving	8	51	2	med
Cappellini, fresh, boiled	301	1 serving	11	57	2	med
Caper sauce, made with semi-skimmed milk	103	5 tbsp	4	10	6	low
Caper sauce, made with skimmed milk	93	5 tbsp	4	10	5	low
Capercaillie, roast	173	¼ bird	31	0	5	0
Capers, pickled	7	1 tbsp	trace	2	0	low
Capon, roast, with skin	216	3 medium slices	23	0	14	0
Capon, roast, without skin	148	3 medium slices	25	0	5	0
Caponata	85	1 slice	3	15	1	med
Cappelletti (stuffed pasta), dried, all stuffings	291 (avge)	1 serving	9	45	6	med
Cappelletti, fresh, all stuffings	229 (avge)	1 serving	9	40	4	med
Cappuccino	101	1 medium cup	2	7	6	0
Capsicum *See* Pepper						
Caramac chocolate bar	170	1 standard bar	2	16	11	0
Caramel ice cream	89	1 scoop	2	12	4	low
Caramel shortcake	171	1 slice	1	20	9	low
Caramel toffees	29	1 toffee	trace	6	1	0
Caramel wafers	113	1 standard bar	1	17	5	low

Food	kCal per portion	Portion size	Protein g	Carbs g	Fat g	Fibre
Carbonara pasta sauce	163	¼ jar	2	5	20	0
Carob bar	470	1 standard bar	7	49	27	high
Carpaccio of beef	61	2 thin slices	10	0	2	0
Carrot	35	1 large carrot	1	8	trace	med
Carrot and orange soup	78	2 ladlefuls	1	12	3	med
Carrot cake	260	1 slice	3	47	7	med
Carrot juice	24	1 small glass	trace	6	trace	0
Carrots, honey-glazed	39	3 heaped tbsp	1	9	trace	med
Carrots, steamed or boiled	24	3 heaped tbsp	1	5	trace	med
Cashew nuts, fresh	143	25 g/1 oz/¼ cup	5	4	12	high
Cashew nuts, roasted	92	1 small handful	3	3	8	high
Cassata	227	1 serving	3	14	23	low
Cassava, baked	310	2 pieces	2	80	trace	high
Cassava, boiled	130	2 pieces	trace	33	trace	high
Cassoulet	341	1 serving	21	38	13	high
Castle pudding	233	1 individual pudding	3	36	2	med
Catfish, fried (sautéed), in breadcrumbs	265	1 piece of fillet	21	9	15	low
Catfish, grilled (broiled)	217	1 piece of fillet	27	0	2	0
Catfish, steamed or poached	141	1 piece of fillet	31	0	2	0
Catsup See Ketchup						
Cauliflower	34	4 med florets	4	3	1	med

Food	kCal per portion	Portion size	Protein g	Carbs g	Fat g	Fibre
Cauliflower, in white sauce, made with semi-skimmed milk	**124**	3 heaped tbsp	6	10	7	med
Cauliflower, in white sauce, made with skimmed milk	**114**	3 heaped tbsp	6	10	6	med
Cauliflower, steamed or boiled	28	4 medium florets	3	2	1	med
Cauliflower bhaji	**150**	1 bhaji	3	3	14	med
Cauliflower cheese	**157**	1 serving	9	8	10	med
Cauliflower soup	**133**	2 ladlefuls	7	16	5	med
Caviar, red or black	**40**	1 tbsp	4	1	3	0
Celeriac (celery root)	**20**	¼ small head	1	3	trace	high
Celeriac, steamed or boiled	**15**	3 heaped tbsp	1	2	trace	high
Celery	**2**	1 stick	trace	trace	trace	low
Celery, braised	**8**	3 heaped tbsp	trace	1	trace	med
Celery root *See* Celeriac						
Celery soup, cream of, canned	**86**	2 ladlefuls	2	7	6	low
Celery soup, packet	**50**	2 ladlefuls	2	8	2	low
Celery soup, home-made	**82**	2 ladlefuls	5	11	2	med
Cellophane noodles, boiled	**251**	1 serving	2	57	trace	low
Ceps mushrooms, stewed	**6**	2 tbsp	1	trace	trace	low
Cereal bars, chewy, all flavours	**131** (avge)	1 bar	1	21	5	med

Food	kCal per portion	Portion size	Protein g	Carbs g	Fat g	Fibre
Cereal bars, crunchy, all flavours	146 (avge)	1 bar	2	17	7	med
Cervelat	77	1 slice	4	trace	7	0
Champagne	114	1 wine glass	trace	2	0	0
Channa dahl	125	3 heaped tbsp	5	10	6	high
Chanterelle mushrooms, stewed	6	2 tbsp	1	trace	trace	low
Chantilly cream	72	1 tbsp	trace	trace	8	0
Chapattis, made with fat	164	1 chapatti	4	24	6	med
Chapattis, made without fat	101	1 chapatti	4	22	trace	med
Charentais melon	57	½ melon	2	13	trace	med
Chargrilled chicken sandwiches	401	1 round	25	29	20	med
Chargrilled chicken breast	192	1 breast	38	0	4	0
Charlotte russe	307	1 serving	6	50	10	low
Chasseur sauce	36	5 tbsp	1	7	trace	0
Chaumes cheese	94	1 small wedge	6	trace	8	0
Cheddar cheese	103	1 small wedge	6	trace	9	0
Cheddar cheese, low-fat	65	1 small wedge	8	trace	4	0
Cheddars	21	1 biscuit (cookie)	trace	2	1	low
Cheerios, dry	92	25 g/1 oz/½ cup	2	18	1	med
Cheerios, with semi-skimmed milk	204	5 heaped tbsp	7	36	3	med

Food	kCal per portion	Portion size	Protein g	Carbs g	Fat g	Fibre
Cheerios, with skimmed milk	**188**	5 heaped tbsp	7	36	1	med
Cheese, fresh, soft, full-fat	**39**	1 heaped tbsp	1	trace	4	0
Cheese, fresh, soft, low-fat	**15**	1 heaped tbsp	1	trace	trace	0
Cheese, fresh, soft, medium-fat	**22**	1 heaped tbsp	1	trace	2	0
Cheese, potted	**267**	1 individual pot	12	1	23	0
See also individual names, e.g. Cheddar						
Cheese and bean enchiladas	**547**	2 enchiladas	28	82	14	high
Cheese and beef enchiladas	**644**	2 enchiladas	24	60	36	low
Cheese and coleslaw sandwiches	**440**	1 round	12	36	28	med
Cheese and ham sandwiches	**432**	1 round	19	34	27	med
Cheese and onion quiche	**396**	1 slice	14	24	28	med
Cheese and pickle sandwiches	**407**	1 round	12	34	26	med
Cheese and pineapple chunks	**25**	1 stick	1	1	2	low
Cheese and tomato pizza, deep-pan	**300**	1 slice	15	30	14	med
Cheese and tomato pizza, thin-crust	**235**	1 slice	9	25	12	med

Food	kCal per portion	Portion size	Protein g	Carbs g	Fat g	Fibre
Cheese and tomato sandwiches	**411**	1 round	13	36	26	med
Cheese fondue	**492**	1 serving	30	8	29	0
Cheese fondue, with French bread bread	**762**	1 serving plus 10 cubes of	40	62	31	low
Cheese footballs	**13**	1 football	trace	1	1	low
Cheese melt biscuits (cookies)	**21**	1 biscuit	trace	3	1	low
Cheese melt biscuits, mini	**6**	1 biscuit	trace	1	trace	low
Cheese omelette	**356**	2 eggs	21	trace	30	0
Cheese on toast	**223**	1 slice	10	21	13	low
Cheese pudding	**292**	1 serving	17	24	14	low
Cheese sandwiches	**398**	1 round	12	34	26	med
Cheese sauce, made with semi-skimmed milk	**134**	5 tbsp	6	7	10	low
Cheese sauce, made with skimmed milk	**124**	5 tbsp	6	7	8	low
Cheese scone (biscuit)	**175**	1 scone	5	21	9	low
Cheese scone, with butter	**249**	1 scone	5	21	17	low
Cheese scone, with low-fat spread	**214**	1 scone	6	21	13	low
Cheese slice, processed	**65**	1 slice	4	trace	5	0
Cheese soufflé	**280**	1 serving	13	10	9	low
Cheese soup, canned	**126**	2 ladlefuls	4	8	8	low

Food	kCal per portion	Portion size	Protein g	Carbs g	Fat g	Fibre
Cheese soup, home-made	94	2 ladlefuls	6	11	3	low
Cheese spread	41	1 tbsp	2	1	3	0
Cheese spread, low-fat	27	1 tbsp	2	1	2	0
Cheese spread, flavoured	35	1 tbsp	2	1	3	low
Cheese straws	28	1 straw	1	2	trace	low
Cheeseburger	299	1 burger in a bun	16	33	11	med
Cheesecake, plain, cooked	490	1 slice	4	30	27	low
Cheesecake, plain, set	272	1 slice	5	30	13	low
Cheesecake, with fruit topping	302	1 slice	7	41	13	low
See also individual flavours, e.g. Chocolate cheesecake						
Cheeselets	147	1 small bag	3	16	8	med
Chelsea bun	329	1 bun	7	50	12	med
Cherries	20	10 cherries	trace	4	trace	low
Cherries, canned in natural juice	51	3 heaped tbsp	trace	13	trace	low
Cherries, canned in syrup	71	3 heaped tbsp	trace	18	trace	low
Cherries, glacé (candied)	13	1 cherry	trace	4	trace	low
Cherries, in brandy/kirsch	126	3 heaped tbsp	trace	18	trace	low
Cherries, maraschino	12	1 cherry	trace	3	trace	low
Cherry bakewells	206	1 individual cake	2	32	8	low
Cherry brandy	64	1 single measure	trace	8	0	0

Food	kCal per portion	Portion size	Protein g	Carbs g	Fat g	Fibre
Cherry cheesecake	302	1 slice	7	41	13	low
Cherry compôte	78	3 heaped tbsp	1	20	trace	low
Cherry genoa cake	334	1 slice	4	51	12	med
Cherry pie	282	1 slice	3	40	13	med
Cherry pie filling	82	¼ large can	trace	21	trace	low
Cherryade	18	1 tumbler	trace	21	trace	0
Cheshire cheese	94	1 small wedge	6	trace	8	0
Chestnut purée, sweetened	45	1 tbsp	trace	10	trace	med
Chestnut purée, unsweetened	25	1 tbsp	trace	5	trace	med
Chestnut stuffing	58	1 serving	1	4	4	med
Chestnuts	18	1 nut	trace	4	trace	high
Chestnuts, peeled and cooked	65	5 nuts	1	14	trace	high
Chestnuts, roasted in shells	21	1 nut	trace	4	trace	high
Chèvre cheese	80	1 small wedge	5	trace	7	0
Chewy cereal bars, all flavours	131 (avge)	1 bar	1	21	5	med
Chick pea dahl	125	3 heaped tbsp	5	10	6	high
Chick pea goulash	338	1 serving	12	36	15	high
Chick peas (garbanzos), canned, drained	115	3 heaped tbsp	7	16	3	high
Chick peas, dried, soaked and boiled	121	3 heaped tbsp	8	18	2	high

Food	kCal per portion	Portion size	Protein g	Carbs g	Fat g	Fibre
Chicken, breast, cooked, sliced	35	1 slice	7	0	1	0
Chicken, breast, grilled (broiled)	213	1 med breast	40	0	6	0
Chicken, breast, poached or steamed	244	1 med breast	44	0	7	0
Chicken, breast, smoked	23	1 slice	2	trace	1	0
Chicken, breast portion, fried (sautéed), in breadcrumbs	363	¼ small chicken	27	22	19	low
Chicken, drumstick, barbecued	103	1 drumstick	16	2	4	0
Chicken, drumstick, roast	92	1 drumstick	15	0	3	0
Chicken, fried	494	2 pieces	36	19	29	low
Chicken, jerk	256	1 serving	32	5	8	trace
Chicken, leg portion, barbecued	287	¼ small chicken	46	1	10	0
Chicken, leg portion, grilled	274	¼ small chicken	46	0	10	0
Chicken, leg portion, roast	276	¼ small chicken	46	0	10	0
Chicken, lemon	356	1 med breast	58	3	13	0
Chicken, minced (ground), stewed	183	1 serving	29	0	7	0
Chicken, roast, with skin	216	3 med slices	23	0	14	0
Chicken, roast, without skin	148	3 med slices	25	0	5	0
Chicken, steamed	197	¼ small chicken	29	7	4	low

Food	kCal per portion	Portion size	Protein g	Carbs g	Fat g	Fibre
Chicken, sweet and sour	165	1 serving	6	32	2	high
Chicken, tandoori	375	¼ small chicken	47	4	19	trace
Chicken, thai, with noodles	506	1 serving	34	59	15	high
Chicken, wing portion, grilled (broiled)	220	¼ small chicken	36	0	9	0
Chicken, wing portion, roast	222	¼ small chicken	36	0	9	0
Chicken, wings, barbecued, Chinese-style	70	1 wing	9	3	2	0
Chicken à la king	255	1 serving	23	20	9	med
Chicken and almond soup, canned	180	2 ladlefuls	5	9	14	low
Chicken and sweetcorn (corn) chowder, home-made	183	2 ladlefuls	25	16	3	med
Chicken and sweetcorn soup, canned	84	2 ladlefuls	3	12	2	low
Chicken and sweetcorn soup, instant	119	1 mug	1	16	6	low
Chicken and ham paste	56	1 tbsp	4	trace	4	0
Chicken and ham pie, cold	380	1 slice	12	32	22	low
Chicken and mushroom casserole	413	1 serving	39	29	16	low
Chicken and mushroom chowder	192	2 ladlefuls	7	17	10	low

Food	kCal per portion	Portion size	Protein g	Carbs g	Fat g	Fibre
Chicken and mushroom pie	**246**	1 individual pie	16	17	12	low
Chicken and mushroom soup, canned	**76**	2 ladlefuls	2	7	4	low
Chicken and mushroom soup, instant	**58**	1 mug	1	9	2	low
Chicken and rice soup, canned	**82**	2 ladlefuls	1	15	2	low
Chicken and rice soup, home-made	**127**	2 ladlefuls	12	13	3	low
Chicken and tarragon soup, home-made	**116**	2 ladlefuls	3	9	8	low
Chicken and vegetable soup, canned	**82**	2 ladlefuls	4	12	2	med
Chicken and vegetable soup,home-made	**165**	2 ladlefuls	12	19	5	high
Chicken and vegetable stir-fry	**270**	1 serving	22	39	7	high
Chicken broth	**64**	2 ladlefuls	2	11	2	low
Chicken burger in a bun, home-made, with relish	**366**	1 burger in a bun	38	32	10	med
Chicken burger sandwich	**710**	1 burger	26	54	43	med
Chicken byriani	**782**	1 serving	18	75	38	med
Chicken cacciatore	**265**	1 serving	22	36	4	high
Chicken casserole	**374**	1 serving	38	29	12	high
Chicken chasseur	**440**	1 serving	27	67	7	med
Chicken chop suey	**295**	1 serving	23	34	6	med

Food	kCal per portion	Portion size	Protein g	Carbs g	Fat g	Fibre
Chicken chow mein	337	1 serving	22	28	5	high
Chicken cordon bleu	344	1 serving	25	15	20	low
Chicken curry, home-made	615	1 serving	31	9	51	med
Chicken curry, home-made, with rice	863	1 serving	36	65	53	med
Chicken curry, retail	447	1 serving	36	16	27	med
Chicken curry, retail, with rice	691	1 serving	37	68	26	high
Chicken enchiladas	566	2 enchiladas	32	66	9	high
Chicken fajitas	258	2 fajitas	16	34	6	low
Chicken fingers	27	1 finger	4	2	1	low
Chicken fricassée	280	1 serving	28	6	16	med
Chicken galantine	268	1 slice	26	9	14	med
Chicken goujons	162	6 goujons	24	12	3	low
Chicken in black bean sauce	221	1 serving	29	10	6	med
Chicken jalfrezi	490	1 serving	26	70	12	high
Chicken kiev	473	1 med breast	28	22	31	low
Chicken korma	460	1 serving	54	16	21	med
Chicken liver pâté	158	1 serving	6	trace	14	0
Chicken liver pâté, with toast and butter	468	1 serving plus 2 slices of toast	13	37	32	med
Chicken liver risotto	590	1 serving	13	89	27	low
Chicken livers, fried (sautéed)	194	1 serving	21	3	11	0

Food	kCal per portion	Portion size	Protein g	Carbs g	Fat g	Fibre
Chicken marsala	**284**	1 serving	27	2	5	low
Chicken maryland	**484**	¼ small chicken	36	30	25	low
Chicken mayonnaise sandwiches	**458**	1 round	12	34	41	med
Chicken noodle soup, canned	**50**	2 ladlefuls	3	8	trace	low
Chicken noodle soup, home-made	**145**	2 ladlefuls	10	17	4	low
Chicken noodle soup, packet	**40**	2 ladlefuls	2	7	1	low
Chicken nuggets	**253**	6 nuggets	19	11	15	med
Chicken omelette	**293**	2 eggs	21	trace	23	0
Chicken paprika	**194**	1 serving	31	6	7	low
Chicken paste	**35**	1 tbsp	2	trace	3	0
Chicken pie, individual	**378**	1 individual pie	12	30	22	low
Chicken pie, with puff pastry (paste)	**572**	1 serving	23	36	37	low
Chicken pot pie	**485**	1 slice	17	28	39	low
Chicken pot roast with vegetables	**510**	1 serving	37	65	11	high
Chicken ravioli	**148**	1 serving	7	26	1	med
Chicken risotto	**336**	1 serving	31	83	8	low
Chicken roll, sliced	**22**	1 slice	3	trace	1	0
Chicken salad	**215**	1 serving	32	5	7	high
Chicken salad, dressed	**318**	1 serving	33	5	19	high
Chicken sandwiches	**341**	1 round	12	34	23	med

Food	kCal per portion	Portion size	Protein g	Carbs g	Fat g	Fibre
Chicken satay	**172**	1 stick	26	6	5	low
Chicken soup, cream of, canned	**116**	2 ladlefuls	3	9	8	0
Chicken soup, home-made	**114**	2 ladlefuls	12	7	4	0
Chicken soup, instant	**100**	1 mug	1	11	6	0
Chicken soup, low-fat, canned	**44**	2 ladlefuls	2	4	2	0
Chicken soup, packet	**128**	2 ladlefuls	2	21	5	0
Chicken stew with dumplings	**537**	1 serving	38	77	9	high
Chicken suprême	**309**	1 breast	43	8	12	low
Chicken tenders	**350**	8 pieces	22	17	22	low
Chicken teriyaki	**317**	1 serving	19	52	4	high
Chicken tikka	**369**	1 serving	43	11	17	med
Chicken tikka masala	**490**	1 serving	38	44	18	high
Chicken véronique	**254**	1 serving	27	11	10	low
Chicken vindaloo	**572**	1 serving	48	7	40	med
Chicory (Belgian endive)	**18**	1 head	2	trace	2	low
Chicory, braised	**38**	1 head	3	2	2	low
Chilli beans	**247**	1 serving	15	52	2	high
Chilli con carne	**302**	1 serving	22	17	17	high
Chilli dog	**204**	1 dog in a bun	7	29	7	low
Chilli salsa	**18**	1 tbsp	trace	4	trace	low
Chilli sauce	**15**	1 tbsp	trace	3	trace	low

Food	kCal per portion	Portion size	Protein g	Carbs g	Fat g	Fibre
Chinese egg noodles, cooked	**124**	1 serving	4	26	1	med
Chinese leaves (stem lettuce)	**11**	1 serving	1	1	0	low
Chinese pork spare ribs	**310**	2 ribs	25	13	17	low
Chipolata sausages, fried (sautéed)	**61**	1 sausage	3	2	5	low
Chipolata sausages, grilled (broiled)	**58**	1 sausage	3	2	5	low
Chips (fries), chip-shop	**394**	1 serving	5	49	20	high
Chips, crinkle-cut, frozen, deep-fried	**478**	1 serving	6	55	27	high
Chips, home-made, deep-fried	**312**	1 serving	6	50	11	high
Chips, microwave	**221**	1 small box	4	32	10	high
Chips, oven, frozen, baked	**267**	1 serving	5	49	7	high
Chips, straight-cut, frozen, deep-fried	**450**	1 serving	6	53	16	high
Chips, thin-cut	**462**	1 serving	5	56	26	high
See also French fries						
Choc ice, any chocolate	**180**	1 ice cream	2	18	11	low
Choco corn flakes, dry	**95**	25 g/1 oz/½ cup	1	21	1	low
Choco corn flakes, with semi-skimmed milk	**209**	5 heaped tbsp	6	35	3	low
Choco corn flakes, with skimmed milk	**193**	5 heaped tbsp	6	35	1	low

Food	kCal per portion	Portion size	Protein g	Carbs g	Fat g	Fibre
Chocolate, milk	255	1 standard bar	4	28	14	0
Chocolate, plain (semi-sweet)	250	1 standard bar	2	30	13	0
Chocolate, white	109	1 standard (thin) bar	2	11	6	0
Chocolate, with fruit and nut	240	1 standard bar	4	27	12	0
Chocolate, with whole nuts	270	1 standard bar	5	24	17	0
Chocolate and walnut brownies	505	1 brownie	7	40	37	med
Chocolate biscuits (cookies), full-coated	131	1 biscuit	1	17	7	low
Chocolate biscuits, half-coated	84	1 biscuit	1	11	4	low
Chocolate brazils	49	1 sweet (candy)	1	3	4	high
Chocolate brownies	368	1 brownie	5	63	11	med
Chocolate buttons	175	1 small packet	3	19	10	0
Chocolate cake, chocolate-coated	268	1 slice	3	41	10	low
Chocolate cake, filled with butter cream	235	1 slice	3	35	10	low
Chocolate caramels	25	1 sweet (candy)	trace	6	trace	low
Chocolate cheesecake	271	1 slice	12	34	11	low
Chocolate chip chewy cereal bar	112	1 bar	1	17	4	low
Chocolate chip cookies	45	1 cookie	trace	8	1	low

Food	kCal per portion	Portion size	Protein g	Carbs g	Fat g	Fibre
Chocolate chip ice cream	91	1 scoop	2	12	4	low
Chocolate chip muffin	397	1 muffin	5	51	22	low
Chocolate corn pops, dry	97	25 g/1 oz/½ cup	1	20	1	low
Chocolate corn pops, with semi-skimmed milk	213	5 heaped tbsp	6	38	4	low
Chocolate corn pops, with skimmed milk	197	5 heaped tbsp	6	38	2	low
Chocolate cream biscuits (cookies)	63	1 biscuit	1	9	3	low
Chocolate cream pie	343	1 slice	3	38	22	low
Chocolate crispix, dry	90	25 g/1 oz/½ cup	1	21	1	low
Chocolate crispix, with semi-skimmed milk	201	5 heaped tbsp	6	40	3	low
Chocolate crispix, with skimmed milk	185	5 heaped tbsp	6	40	1	low
Chocolate custard, canned	71	¼ large can	2	11	2	low
Chocolate dessert	136	1 individual pot	2	19	5	low
Chocolate dessert, with cream	225	1 individual pot	4	24	12	low
Chocolate digestives (graham crackers)	88	1 biscuit (cookie)	1	11	4	med
Chocolate éclair toffees	48	1 toffee	trace	7	2	low
Chocolate éclair, filled with cream	277	1 éclair	4	18	21	low

Food	kCal per portion	Portion size	Protein g	Carbs g	Fat g	Fibre
Chocolate éclair, filled with custard	**262**	1 éclair	6	24	16	low
Chocolate finger biscuits (cookies)	**38**	1 biscuit	trace	5	2	low
Chocolate fudge	**65**	1 piece	trace	13	1	low
Chocolate fudge cake	**420**	1 slice	5	70	14	low
Chocolate fudge fingers	**135**	1 finger	1	22	5	0
Chocolate fudge icing (frosting)	**77**	1 tbsp	trace	9	1	low
Chocolate ginger	**30**	1 piece	trace	7	trace	low
Chocolate ice cream	**89**	1 scoop	2	12	4	low
Chocolate layer cake	**384**	1 slice	5	58	14	low
Chocolate mini roll	**119**	1 roll	1	16	5	low
Chocolate mint creams	**39**	1 mint	trace	8	1	0
Chocolate mousse	**139**	1 individual pot	4	10	5	0
Chocolate mousse, low-calorie	**88**	1 individual pot	0	0	3	0
Chocolate nut sundae	**417**	1 sundae	4	52	23	low
Chocolate peanuts	**200**	1 small packet	5	19	13	med
Chocolate pot	**136**	1 individual pot	2	19	5	low
Chocolate profiteroles	**373**	1 serving	6	33	24	med
Chocolate pudding	**340**	1 serving	6	45	16	med
Chocolate raisins	**185**	1 small packet	2	32	7	high
Chocolate ripple ice-cream	**89**	1 scoop	2	12	4	low
Chocolate roulade	**206**	1 serving	4	20	12	0

Food	kCal per portion	Portion size	Protein g	Carbs g	Fat g	Fibre
Chocolate sauce, for ice cream	**192**	2 tbsp	5	29	6	low
Chocolate sauce, made with semi-skimmed milk	**112**	5 tbsp	3	14	5	low
Chocolate sauce, made with skimmed milk	**102**	5 tbsp	3	14	4	low
Chocolate shreddies, dry	**91**	25 g/1 oz/½ cup	2	20	trace	med
Chocolate shreddies, with semi-skimmed milk	**224**	5 heaped tbsp	8	42	3	high
Chocolate shreddies, with skimmed milk	**208**	5 heaped tbsp	8	42	1	high
Chocolate soufflé	**103**	1 serving	7	17	1	low
Chocolate soya ice dessert	**52**	1 scoop	1	5	3	0
Chocolate spread, all types	**82** (avge)	1 tbsp	1	9	5	low
Chocolate spread, with peanut butter	**89**	1 tbsp	2	5	7	med
Chocolate wafer bar	**115**	1 standard bar	1	13	6	0
Chocolates, assorted, filled	**46** (avge)	1 chocolate	trace	7	2	0
Chorizo sausage	**273**	1 small sausage	14	1	23	0
Choux buns, filled with cream	**237**	1 bun	4	8	21	low
Choux buns, filled with custard	**293**	1 bun	7	27	17	low

Food	kCal per portion	Portion size	Protein g	Carbs g	Fat g	Fibre
Christmas cake, with marzipan and royal icing (frosting)	**356**	1 slice	4	63	11	med
Christmas pudding	**291**	1 serving	5	49	10	med
Ciabatta bread	**125**	1 med slice	4	26	trace	med
Cider, dry	**108**	1 small	trace	8	0	0
Cider, med-sweet	**126**	1 small	trace	13	0	0
Cider, vintage	**303**	1 small	trace	22	0	0
Cider cup	**62**	1 wine glass	trace	17	0	0
Cigarettes russes	**56**	1 biscuit (cookie)	1	6	3	low
Cinnamon danish pastries	**270**	1 pastry	6	52	18	med
Cinnamon grahams, dry	**102**	25 g/1 oz/½ cup	1	19	2	med
Cinnamon grahams, with semi-skimmed milk	**182**	3 heaped tbsp	5	29	5	med
Cinnamon grahams, with skimmed milk	**166**	3 heaped tbsp	5	29	3	med
Clafoutis	**242**	1 serving	7	33	10	med
Clam bisque, canned	**85**	2 ladlefuls	5	12	2	low
Clam chowder, home-made	**253**	2 ladlefuls	22	17	10	med
Clams, canned, drained	**60**	½ medium can	9	2	1	0
Clams, fresh, shelled, cooked	**93**	1 serving	15	4	1	0
Classic chocolate bar	**125**	1 standard bar	1	15	7	low

Food	kCal per portion	Portion size	Protein g	Carbs g	Fat g	Fibre
Clear conserve *See* Jelly, *individual flavours*, *e.g.* Mint jelly, Redcurrant jelly						
Clementine	**28**	1 fruit	1	6	trace	med
Clotted cream fudge	**80**	1 square	trace	14	3	0
Club chocolate bar, all flavours	**125** (avge)	1 bar	1	16	7	low
Clusters, dry	**97**	25 g/1 oz/½ cup	3	17	2	med
Clusters, with skimmed milk	**160**	3 heaped tbsp	7	26	3	med
Clusters, with semi-skimmed milk	**176**	3 heaped tbsp	7	26	5	med
Cob loaf	**70**	1 med slice	3	15	1	low
Cob nuts, shelled	**162**	25 g/1 oz/¼ cup	3	1	16	med
Cobbler *See individual flavours, e.g.* Fruit cobbler						
Coca-cola	**78**	1 tumbler	trace	21	0	0
Coca-cola, diet	**1**	1 tumbler	0	0	0	0
Cock-a-leekie soup, home-made	**138**	2 ladlefuls	2	15	8	low
Cockles, fresh, shelled, cooked	**48**	1 serving	11	trace	trace	0
Cockles, preserved in vinegar	**49**	1 serving	12	1	trace	0
Cocktail sauce	**51**	1 tbsp	trace	2	4	low
Coco pops, dry	**95**	25 g/1 oz/½ cup	1	21	1	low

Food	kCal per portion	Portion size	Protein g	Carbs g	Fat g	Fibre
Coco pops, with semi-skimmed milk	**209**	5 heaped tbsp	5	27	3	low
Coco pops, with skimmed milk	**193**	5 heaped tbsp	5	27	1	low
Coco pops cereal and milk bar	**90**	1 bar	2	14	3	low
Cocoa, made with semi-skimmed milk and sugar	**142**	1 mug	9	17	5	low
Cocoa, made with skimmed milk and sugar	**126**	1 mug	9	17	3	low
Coconut	**330**	¼ nut	3	13	31	high
Coconut, desiccated (shredded)	**43**	1 tbsp	1	1	9	high
Coconut cake	**175**	1 slice	3	20	19	low
Coconut ice sweet (candy) bar	**464**	1 standard bar	2	83	13	high
Coconut macaroons	**117**	1 macaroon	1	16	5	med
Coconut pyramid	**230**	1 pyramid	1	42	6	high
Coconut rings/thins	**35**	1 biscuit (cookie)	trace	5	1	low
Cod, baked	**168**	1 piece of fillet	37	0	2	0
Cod, grilled (broiled)	**166**	1 piece of fillet	36	0	2	0
Cod, fried (sautéed), in batter	**497**	1 piece of fillet	49	19	26	low
Cod, fried (sautéed), in breadcrumbs	**435**	1 piece of fillet	53	9	21	low
Cod, salt, soaked and cooked	**241**	1 piece of fillet	57	0	2	0
Cod, with butter sauce	**159**	1 steak	18	9	9	low

Food	kCal per portion	Portion size	Protein g	Carbs g	Fat g	Fibre
Cod, with cheese sauce	175	1 steak	20	9	6	low
Cod, with mushroom sauce	168	1 steak	18	9	8	low
Cod, with parsley sauce	170	1 steak	19	11	5	low
Cod and prawn pie	328	1 individual pie	17	24	21	low
Cod mornay	415	1 steak	29	23	23	low
Cod provençal	273	1 serving	39	9	9	med
Cod roes, in breadcrumbs, fried (sautéed)	202	1 serving	21	3	12	low
Cod roes, on toast	307	1 serving plus 1 slice of toast	20	10	20	low
Coffee, black	5	1 mug	trace	1	trace	0
Coffee, espresso	4	1 small cup	trace	1	trace	0
Coffee, white, made with water and semi-skimmed milk	15	1 mug	1	2	trace	0
Coffee, white, made with water and skimmed milk	12	1 mug	1	2	trace	0
Coffee and walnut cake	344	1 slice	7	34	19	med
Coffee cake	258	1 slice	5	34	11	low
Coffee cheesecake	272	1 slice	5	30	13	low
Coffee granita	44	1 serving	trace	11	trace	0
Coffee ice cream	89	1 scoop	2	12	4	low
Coffee mousse	139	1 serving	4	20	5	0
Coffee roulade	206	1 slice	4	20	12	0

Food	kCal per portion	Portion size	Protein g	Carbs g	Fat g	Fibre
Coffee streusel cake	263	1 slice	4	29	15	med
Coffeemate	27	1 tsp	trace	3	2	0
Coffeemate, light	21	1 tsp	trace	3	1	0
Cointreau	78	1 single measure	trace	7	0	0
Cola	78	1 tumbler	trace	21	0	0
Cola, low-calorie	1	1 tumbler	0	0	0	0
Colcannon	240	1 serving	3	7	18	high
Coleslaw, home-made	92	2 tbsp	3	13	4	high
Coleslaw, low-calorie	28	2 tbsp	trace	2	2	med
Coleslaw, ready-made	40	2 tbsp	trace	3	3	med
Coley, fried (sautéed), in batter	490	1 piece of fillet	48	19	25	low
Coley, fried, in breadcrumbs	428	1 piece of fillet	52	9	20	low
Coley, poached or steamed	147	1 piece of fillet	35	0	1	0
Collard greens *See* Spring greens						
Complan, savoury, made with water	194	1 mug	10	24	7	0
Complan, sweet, made withsemi-skimmed milk	260	1 mug	14	34	9	low
Complan, sweet, made with skimmed milk	240	1 mug	14	34	6	low
Complan, sweet, made with water	192	1 mug	9	27	6	low

Food	kCal per portion	Portion size	Protein g	Carbs g	Fat g	Fibre
Conchiglie (pasta shapes), dried, boiled	**198**	1 serving	7	42	1	med
Conchiglie, fresh, boiled	**235**	1 serving	9	45	2	med
Condensed milk, skimmed, sweetened	**267**	100 ml/3½ fl oz/ scant ½ cup	10	60	trace	0
Condensed milk, skimmed, unsweetened	**80**	100 ml/3½ fl oz/ scant ½ cup	10	11	trace	0
Condensed milk, whole, sweetened	**333**	100 ml/3½ fl oz/ scant ½ cup	8	55	10	0
Condensed milk, whole, unsweetened	**151**	100 ml/3½ fl oz/ scant ½ cup	8	8	9	0
Conger eel, grilled (broiled)	**375**	1 steak	38	0	24	0
Consommé, canned	**14**	2 ladlefuls	3	1	trace	0
Consommé, jellied	**32**	2 ladlefuls	5	2	trace	0
Cookies See Biscuits						
Cook-in sauces, all flavours	**43** (avge)	1 serving	1	8	1	low
Coq au vin	**410**	1 serving	30	7	29	low
Coquilles st jacques	**212**	1 serving	10	20	10	med
Cordial See individual flavours, e.g. Blackcurrant cordial						
Corn chips	**229**	1 small bag	4	30	11	med
Corn chowder	**143**	2 ladlefuls	5	28	2	high
Corn cobs, baby, canned, drained	**23**	4 cobs	3	2	trace	med

Food	kCal per portion	Portion size	Protein g	Carbs g	Fat g	Fibre
Corn cobs, baby, steamed or boiled	**24**	4 cobs	2	3	trace	med
Corn cobs, baby, stir-fried	**69**	4 cobs	2	3	5	med
Corn flakes, dry	**92**	25 g/1 oz/½ cup	2	20	trace	low
Corn flakes, with semi-skimmed milk	**149**	5 heaped tbsp	6	27	2	low
Corn flakes, with skimmed milk	**133**	5 heaped tbsp	6	27	trace	low
Corn flakes cereal and chocolate milk bar	**118**	1 bar	2	18	4	low
Corn fritters	**91**	1 fritter	2	16	2	med
Corn kernels, canned, drained *See also* Sweetcorn	**122**	3 heaped tbsp	3	27	1	med
Corn pops, dry	**90**	25 g/1 oz/½ cup	1	22	trace	low
Corn pops, with semi-skimmed milk	**209**	5 heaped tbsp	7	38	3	low
Corn pops, with skimmed milk	**193**	5 heaped tbsp	7	38	1	low
Corn pops, chocolate, dry	**97**	25 g/1 oz/½ cup	1	20	1	low
Corn pops, chocolate, with semi-skimmed milk	**213**	5 heaped tbsp	6	38	4	low
Corn pops, chocolate, with skimmed milk	**197**	5 heaped tbsp	6	38	2	low
Corn puff snacks, all flavours	**259** (avge)	1 small bag	3	27	16	low

Food	kCal per portion	Portion size	Protein g	Carbs g	Fat g	Fibre
Corn salad	3	1 handful	trace	trace	trace	low
Cornbread	153	1 piece	4	22	5	med
Corned beef	54	1 slice	7	0	3	0
Corned beef hash	387	1 serving	21	22	24	med
Cornetto, all flavours	198 (avge)	1 cornet	3	26	10	low
Cornflour pudding	134	1 serving	6	26	2	low
Cornichons *See* Gherkins						
Cornish crab soup, canned	118	2 ladlefuls	6	25	trace	low
Cornish hen *See* Poussin						
Cornish ice cream	80	1 scoop	1	6	2	0
Cornish pasties	515	1 pasty	12	48	32	med
Cornish wafers	47	1 wafer	1	5	3	low
Cornmeal *See* Polenta						
Cornmeal muffins	154	1 muffin	4	23	6	low
Cornmeal pancakes	97	1 pancake	3	15	3	low
Corn on the cob, steamed or boiled	99	1 cob	4	17	2	med
Corn on the cob, with butter	173	1 cob	4	17	10	med
Corn on the cob, with low-fat spread	138	1 cob	4	17	6	med
Coronation chicken	266	1 serving	40	15	5	low
Cottage cheese	98	1 small tub	14	2	4	0

Food	kCal per portion	Portion size	Protein g	Carbs g	Fat g	Fibre
Cottage cheese, flavoured	**95**	1 small tub	13	3	4	0
Cottage cheese, low-fat	**78**	1 small tub	13	3	1	0
Cottage cheese, low-fat, flavoured	**75**	1 small tub	12	3	1	0
Cottage loaf	**74**	1 med slice	3	15	1	low
Cottage pie	**330**	1 serving	24	25	19	med
Coulibiac	**380**	1 thick slice	12	30	25	low
Country store, dry	**87**	25 g/1 oz/¼ cup	2	17	1	med
Country store, with semi-skimmed milk	**197**	3 heaped tbsp	8	33	4	high
Country store, with skimmed milk	**181**	3 heaped tbsp	8	33	2	high
Courgettes (zucchini), fried (sautéed)	**63**	3 heaped tbsp	3	3	5	med
Courgettes, steamed or boiled	**19**	3 heaped tbsp	2	2	trace	med
Courgettes, stuffed	**134**	2 halves	5	12	8	med
Courgettes provençal	**69**	3 heaped tbsp	3	8	3	med
Couscous	**177**	3 heaped tbsp	6	29	4	med
Couscous salad	**159**	3 heaped tbsp	5	23	6	high
Crab, dressed	**459**	1 med crab	63	17	16	low
Crab, dressed, canned	**21**	½ small can	3	0	3	0
Crab, white meat	**81**	½ small can	18	0	1	0
Crab and mayonnaise sandwiches	**447**	1 round	15	34	29	med

Food	kCal per portion	Portion size	Protein g	Carbs g	Fat g	Fibre
Crab bisque, home-made	**185**	2 ladlefuls	6	26	7	low
Crab cakes	**93**	1 cake	12	trace	4	0
Crab cocktail	**102**	1 serving	10	7	3	med
Crab sandwiches	**344**	1 round	14	34	18	med
Crabapple jelly (clear conserve)	**55**	1 tbsp	trace	13	trace	0
Crabsticks	**12**	1 stick	2	1	trace	0
Cracked wheat *See* Bulgar						
Crackerbread	**20**	1 piece	trace	4	trace	low
Crackers, wholemeal *See also Biscuits and individual names, e.g.* Ritz	**29**	1 cracker	1	5	1	med
Cranberries, dried	**48**	1 small handful	trace	12	trace	high
Cranberries, stewed with sugar	**70**	3 heaped tbsp	trace	18	trace	low
Cranberry jelly (clear conserve)	**38**	1 tbsp	trace	10	0	low
Cranberry juice drink	**104**	1 tumbler	trace	25	0	0
Cranberry juice drink, light	**48**	1 tumbler	trace	11	0	0
Cranberry sauce	**24**	1 tbsp	trace	6	0	low
Crayfish, boiled	148	½ crayfish	30	0	2	0
Cream, aerosol	**46**	1 tbsp	trace	trace	5	0
Cream, canned	**36**	1 tbsp	trace	trace	4	0

Food	kCal per portion	Portion size	Protein g	Carbs g	Fat g	Fibre
Cream, clotted	88	1 tbsp	trace	trace	9	0
Cream, double (heavy)	67	1 tbsp	trace	trace	7	0
Cream, half	22	1 tbsp	trace	1	2	0
Cream, single (light)	30	1 tbsp	trace	1	3	0
Cream, soured (dairy sour)	31	1 tbsp	trace	1	3	0
Cream, sweetened, imitation	28	1 tbsp	trace	1	4	0
Cream, whipping	56	1 tbsp	trace	trace	6	0
Cream cake	337	1 individual cake	6	43	17	low
Cream cheese	110	1 heaped tbsp	1	trace	12	0
Cream crackers	39	1 cracker	1	6	1	low
Cream crowdie	691	1 serving	3	14	52	med
Cream of wheat See Semolina						
Cream soda	58	1 tumbler	trace	14	trace	low
Cream soups, canned, all flavours See also individual entries, e.g. Cream of tomato soup	110 (avge)	2 ladlefuls	2	9	8	low
Crème brûlée	492	1 serving	1	18	50	0
Crème caramel	136	1 individual pot	4	26	2	0
Crème de cassis	65	1 single measure	trace	7	0	0
Crème de menthe	125	1 single measure	0	14	trace	0
Creme egg, chocolate	163	1 egg	2	28	6	0
Crème fraîche	56	1 tbsp	trace	trace	6	0

Food	kCal per portion	Portion size	Protein g	Carbs g	Fat g	Fibre
Crème fraîche, low-fat	**25**	1 tbsp	trace	1	2	0
Crêpe, plain	**122**	1 crêpe	2	14	7	low
Crêpes suzette	**317**	2 pancakes	4	28	12	med
Crispbread, rye	**27**	1 cracker	1	6	trace	med
Crispbread, starch-reduced	**15**	1 cracker	trace	3	trace	low
Crispbread, wheat	**35**	1 cracker	1	7	trace	low
Crispie cakes	**69**	1 cake	1	11	3	low
Crisps (potato chips), all flavours	**136** (avge)	1 small bag	1	12	9	med
Crisps, low-fat, all flavours	**114** (avge)	1 small bag	2	16	5	med
Crispy chicken sandwich	**500**	1 portion	23	54	27	med
Crispy chicken strips	**300**	3 strips	26	18	16	low
Crispy duck with pancakes	**665**	1 serving plus 6 pancakes	39	32	42	high
Crispy noodles	**374**	1 serving	4	50	17	low
Crispy vegetable fingers	**45**	1 finger	1	5	2	low
Croissant, all-butter	**185**	1 croissant	4	20	10	low
Croissant, apple	**144**	1 croissant	4	21	5	med
Croissant, chocolate	**236**	1 croissant	4	26	13	low
Croissant, mini	**140**	1 croissant	3	15	8	low
Croissant, raisin	**212**	1 croissant	4	27	10	med
Croque monsieur	**438**	1 round	20	36	27	med
Croquette potatoes, fried (sautéed)	**214**	2 croquettes	4	22	13	med

Food	kCal per portion	Portion size	Protein g	Carbs g	Fat g	Fibre
Croquette potatoes, frozen, baked	90	2 croquettes	2	14	3	low
Crostini, garlic	31	1 slice	1	5	1	low
Crostini, mushroom	92	1 slice	3	16	2	low
Croûtons	75	1 tbsp	1	7	5	low
Crown roast of lamb	488	2 cutlets	30	0	40	0
Crudités	35	1 good handful	1	8	0	med
Crudités, with aioli	272	1 serving	1	8	23	med
Crumpet	80	1 crumpet	3	10	0	low
Crumpet, toasted, with butter	117	1 crumpet	3	10	4	low
Crumpet, toasted, with low-fat spread	99	1 crumpet	4	10	2	low
Crunchie chocolate bar	195	1 standard bar	2	30	8	0
Crunchy bran, dry	74	25 g/1 oz/½ cup	3	13	1	high
Crunchy bran, with semi-skimmed milk	175	5 heaped tbsp	9	27	4	high
Crunchy bran, with skimmed milk	159	5 heaped tbsp	9	27	2	high
Crunchy cereal bars, all flavours	146 (avge)	1 bar	2	17	7	med
Crunchy mixed grain cereal, with nuts and raisins, dry	97	25 g/1 oz/¼ cup	2	16	3	high
Crunchy mixed grain cereal, with nuts and raisins andsemi-skimmed milk	250	3 heaped tbsp	9	37	7	high

Food	kCal per portion	Portion size	Protein g	Carbs g	Fat g	Fibre
Crunchy mixed grain cereal, with nuts and raisins and skimmed milk	234	3 heaped tbsp	9	37	5	high
Crunchy nut corn flakes, dry	97	25 g/1 oz/½ cup	2	20	1	low
Crunchy nut corn flakes, with semi-skimmed milk	213	5 heaped tbsp	7	39	3	low
Crunchy nut corn flakes, with skimmed milk	197	5 heaped tbsp	7	39	1	low
Cucumber	4	5 slices	0	1	0	low
Cucumber and yoghurt soup	78	2 ladlefuls	5	9	3	low
Cucumber sandwiches	308	1 round	5	35	17	med
Cullen skink	170	2 ladlefuls	13	16	6	low
Cumberland butter	53	1 tbsp	0	29	22	0
Cumberland sauce	64	1 tbsp	trace	14	trace	0
Cumberland sausage, fried (sautéed)	317	1 sausage	14	11	24	low
Cupcakes, iced (frosted)	179	1 cake	1	37	3	low
Curaçao	78	1 single measure	trace	7	0	0
Curd cheese	30	1 heaped tbsp	4	trace	12	0
Curd, lemon or orange	42	1 tbsp	trace	9	1	low
Curly endive (frisée)	6	1 good handful	trace	2	trace	med
Curly kale, steamed or boiled	24	3 heaped tbsp	2	1	1	med

Food	kCal per portion	Portion size	Protein g	Carbs g	Fat g	Fibre
Curly wurly chocolate bar	**125**	1 standard bar	1	20	5	0
Currant bread	**72**	1 slice	2	13	2	low
Currant bread, with butter	**146**	1 slice	2	13	10	low
Currant bread, with low-fat spread	**111**	1 slice	3	13	6	low
Currant bun	**148**	1 bun	4	26	4	med
Currant bun, with butter	**222**	1 bun	4	26	12	med
Currant bun, with low-fat spread	**187**	1 bun	4	26	8	med
Currant cake	**177**	1 slice	2	29	6	med
Currants	**40**	1 small handful	trace	10	trace	high
Curried beans	**168**	1 small can	10	31	1	high
Curried chicken and rice salad	**390**	1 serving	42	43	6	high
Curried fruit chutney	**19**	1 tbsp	trace	4	trace	low
Curry sauce	**58**	5 tbsp	1	5	4	low
Custard, canned/carton	**71**	5 tbsp	2	11	2	low
Custard, chocolate	**71**	5 tbsp	2	11	2	low
Custard, egg, baked	**130**	1 serving	6	12	7	0
Custard, made with powder and semi-skimmed milk	**75**	5 tbsp	3	13	trace	low
Custard, made with powder and skimmed milk	**59**	5 tbsp	3	13	2	low

Food	kCal per portion	Portion size	Protein g	Carbs g	Fat g	Fibre
Custard apple	101	1 fruit	2	25	1	med
Custard creams	57	1 biscuit (cookie)	1	8	3	low
Custard sauce, made with semi-skimmed milk	62	5 tbsp	2	7	2	0
Custard sauce, made with skimmed milk	52	5 tbsp	2	7	1	0
Custard tart	373	1 individual tart	8	44	20	med
Custard-style yoghurt	161	1 individual pot	8	3	13	0
Cuttlefish, grilled (broiled)	278	1 serving	56	2	2	0

Food	kCal per portion	Portion size	Protein g	Carbs g	Fat g	Fibre
Dab, fried (sautéed) in breadcrumbs	**378**	1 medium fish	28	16	23	low
Dab, grilled (broiled)	**175**	1 medium fish	35	0	3	0
Daiquiri	**111**	1 cocktail	trace	4	0	0
Dairy milk chocolate bar	**255**	1 standard bar	4	28	14	0
Daktyla bread	**65**	1 medium slice	2	12	1	med
Damsons	**3**	1 fruit	trace	1	trace	med
Damsons, stewed	**27**	3 heaped tbsp	1	6	trace	med
Damsons, stewed with sugar	**107**	3 heaped tbsp	1	19	trace	med
Damson jam (conserve)	**39**	1 tbsp	trace	10	0	0
Damson pie	**290**	1 slice	3	14	39	med
Dandelion and burdock	**56**	1 tumbler	0	13	trace	low
Dandelion and burdock, low-calorie	**3**	1 tumbler	0	0	0	0
Danish apple cake	**252**	1 slice	3	32	10	high
Danish blue cheese	**87**	1 small wedge	5	trace	7	0
Danish brown bread	**51**	1 medium slice	2	10	trace	med
Danish elbo cheese	**86**	1 small wedge	6	trace	7	0
Danish lumpfish roe	**40**	1 tbsp	4	1	3	0
Danish pastries, all types	**374** (avge)	1 pastry	6	51	18	med
Danish toaster bread	**65**	1 slice	2	12	1	low
Danish toaster bread, toasted, with butter	**129**	1 slice	2	12	9	low

Food	kCal per portion	Portion size	Protein g	Carbs g	Fat g	Fibre
Danish toaster bread, toasted, with low-fat spread	94	1 slice	2	12	5	low
Danish white bread	50	1 medium slice	2	10	trace	low
Date squares	170	1 square	4	32	4	high
Dates	30	1 fruit	trace	8	trace	high
Dates, dried	40	1 fruit	trace	10	trace	high
Dates, stuffed	50	1 fruit	2	12	4	high
Dauphinoise potatoes	235	1 serving	14	12	15	med
Derby cheese	100	1 small wedge	6	trace	8	0
Devilled chicken	309	1 serving	48	6	12	0
Devilled kidneys	158	1 serving	21	2	7	0
Devil's food cake	255	1 slice	3	40	8	low
Devils on horseback	52	1 roll	1	3	4	low
Dhal	162	3 heaped tbsp	7	21	6	high
Diet coke	1	1 tumbler	0	0	0	0
Diet pepsi	1	1 tumbler	trace	trace	trace	0
Digestive biscuits (graham crackers)	73	1 biscuit (cookie)	1	10	3	low
Digestive caramels, chocolate	81	1 biscuit	1	11	4	med
Digestive creams	63	1 biscuit (cookie)	1	8	3	low
Dijon mustard	8	1 tsp	trace	trace	trace	low
Dill pickled cucumbers	15	1 pickle	trace	3	trace	low

Food	kCal per portion	Portion size	Protein g	Carbs g	Fat g	Fibre
Dim sum, assorted	**49** (avge)	1 piece	3	6	2	low
Ditali (pasta shapes), dried, boiled	**198**	1 serving	7	42	1	med
Ditali, fresh, boiled	**235**	1 serving	9	45	2	med
Dogfish, fried (sautéed), in batter	**464**	1 piece of fillet	29	13	33	low
Dolcelatte cheese	**106**	1 small wedge	4	trace	10	0
Dolmas	**221**	2 rolls	18	19	9	high
Donor kebab, in pitta bread	**588**	1 kebab plus 1 bread	33	32	38	med
Dorset blue cheese	**87**	1 small wedge	5	trace	7	0
Double chocolate chip muffin	**397**	1 muffin	5	48	20	low
Double decker chocolate bar	**235**	1 bar	3	32	10	0
Double gloucester cheese	**101**	1 small wedge	6	trace	8	0
Doughnut, apple	**243**	1 doughnut	4	29	12	low
Doughnut, chocolate	**270**	1 doughnut	3	26	18	med
Doughnut, cream	**265**	1 doughnut	4	43	15	low
Doughnut, iced (frosted)	**286**	1 doughnut	4	42	12	low
Doughnut, jam (jelly)	**252**	1 doughnut	4	37	11	low
Doughnut, mini	**59**	1 doughnut	1	7	3	low
Doughnut, plain, ring	**236**	1 doughnut	4	27	12	low

Food	kCal per portion	Portion size	Protein g	Carbs g	Fat g	Fibre
Dover sole, fried (sautéed), in seasoned flour	342	1 medium fish	25	8	13	low
Dover sole, grilled (broiled)	202	1 medium fish	29	0	9	0
Dr pepper soft drink	78	1 tumbler	trace	21	0	0
Dr pepper, diet	1	1 tumbler	0	0	0	0
Drambuie	85	1 single measure	trace	7	0	0
Dream topping, made with semi-skimmed milk	75	3 heaped tbsp	2	5	6	low
Dream topping, made with skimmed milk	66	3 heaped tbsp	2	5	4	low
Dream topping, sugar-free, made with semi-skimmed milk	75	3 heaped tbsp	3	5	5	low
Dream topping, sugar-free, made with skimmed milk	70	3 heaped tbsp	3	5	3	0
Dressed crab	459	1 medium crab	63	17	16	low
Dressed crab, canned	21	½ small can	3	0	3	0
Dried fruit compôte	127	3 heaped tbsp	2	33	trace	high
Drifter chocolate bar	292	1 standard bar	3	40	13	low
Drinking (sweetened) chocolate, made with semi-skimmed milk	177	1 mug	9	27	5	low
Drinking chocolate, made with skimmed milk	146	1 mug	9	27	1	low

Food	kCal per portion	Portion size	Protein g	Carbs g	Fat g	Fibre
Drinking chocolate, instant, made with water	119	1 mug	3	18	4	low
Drinking yoghurt	124	1 tumbler	6	26	trace	0
Drop scone (small pancake)	44	1 pancake	1	6	2	low
Dry-cured Belgian ham	21	1 slice	4	0	1	0
Dry-roasted peanuts	88	1 small handful	4	1	7	high
Dublin bay prawns (saltwater crayfish), cooked	10	1 prawn	2	0	trace	0
Dubonnet, red	75	1 double measure	trace	8	0	0
Duchesse potatoes	165	2 pieces	5	17	5	med
Duck, breast, grilled (broiled), without skin	378	1 breast	50	0	19	0
Duck, breast, grilled, with skin	678	1 breast	37	0	58	0
Duck, crispy peking	665	1 serving plus 6 pancakes	39	32	42	high
Duck, roast, with skin	763	¼ duck	44	0	65	0
Duck à l'orange	856	¼ duck	49	8	69	med
Duck eggs, boiled	106	1 egg	9	trace	8	0
Duck liver pâté	158	1 serving	6	trace	14	0
Duck soup, home-made	114	2 ladlefuls	12	7	4	0
Duck with cherries	836	¼ duck	44	4	65	low
Dumplings	73	1 dumpling	1	9	1	low
Dundee cake	397	1 slice	6	58	17	med

Food	kCal per portion	Portion size	Protein g	Carbs g	Fat g	Fibre
Dunlop cheese	**103**	1 small wedge	6	trace	9	0
Dutch apple tart	**237**	1 slice	3	34	10	med

Food	kCal per portion	Portion size	Protein g	Carbs g	Fat g	Fibre
Easter biscuits (cookies)	58	1 biscuit	1	16	4	low
Eccles cake	214	1 cake	2	26	12	med
Echo chocolate bar	132	1 standard bar	2	15	7	low
Eclair, chocolate	277	1 éclair	4	18	21	low
Edam (dutch) cheese	83	1 small wedge	6	trace	6	0
Eel pie mash, with pea gravy	434	1 serving	17	35	25	med
Eels, jellied	70	1 small serving	6	trace	6	0
Eels, silver, stewed	320	1 serving	25	0	13	0
Eels, smoked	167	1 serving	10	0	13	0
Egg, baked, with cream	151	1 egg	7	trace	13	0
Egg, boiled	84	1 egg	7	trace	6	0
Egg, coddled	84	1 egg	7	trace	6	0
Egg, curried	226	2 eggs	15	5	16	low
Egg, fried (sautéed)	102	1 egg	8	trace	8	0
Egg, pickled	84	1 egg	7	trace	6	0
Egg, poached	84	1 egg	7	trace	6	0
Egg, scotch	301	1 egg	14	16	20	low
Egg, scrambled	308	2 eggs	13	1	28	0
Egg, stuffed	187	2 halves	7	trace	17	0
Egg and cress sandwiches	392	1 round	13	68	23	med
Egg custard tart	373	1 individual tart	8	44	20	med
Egg custard, baked	130	1 serving	6	12	7	0

Food	kCal per portion	Portion size	Protein g	Carbs g	Fat g	Fibre
Egg custard, packet, made up with semi-skimmed milk	**168**	1 serving	5	23	6	0
Egg custard, packet, made up with skimmed milk	**149**	1 serving	5	23	4	0
Egg fried rice	**374**	1 serving	7	46	19	low
Egg mayonnaise	**290**	1 egg	7	trace	29	0
Egg mayonnaise sandwiches	**491**	1 round	13	34	34	med
Egg mcmuffin	**290**	1 portion	17	27	12	med
Egg nog	**68**	1 single measure	1	7	2	0
Egg noodles, chinese	**124**	1 serving	4	26	1	med
Egg salad	**200**	2 eggs	16	5	12	high
Egg salad, dressed	**297**	2 eggs	16	5	29	high
Egg sauce	**117**	5 tbsp	5	8	7	low
Eggplant See Aubergine						
Eggs benedict	**402**	1 egg	22	43	17	med
Eggs florentine	**239**	1 egg	16	7	16	med
Eggy bread	**213**	1 slice	6	17	18	low
Elderflower pressé	**50**	1 wine glass	trace	12	trace	0
Elmlea cream blend, double (heavy)	**61**	1 tbsp	trace	trace	6	low
Elmlea, single (light)	**48**	1 tbsp	trace	trace	5	low
Elmlea, whipping	**43**	1 tbsp	trace	trace	4	low
Elmlea light, double (heavy)	**37**	1 tbsp	trace	1	4	low

Food	kCal per portion	Portion size	Protein g	Carbs g	Fat g	Fibre
Elmlea light, single (light)	17	1 tbsp	trace	trace	3	low
Elmlea light, whipping	28	1 tbsp	trace	trace	2	low
Emmental (swiss) cheese	105	1 small wedge	7	1	8	0
Enchiladas See individual fillings, e.g. Cheese enchiladas						
English muffin	127	1 muffin	5	27	1	med
English muffin, toasted, with butter	200	1 muffin	5	27	9	med
English muffin, toasted, with low-fat spread	166	1 muffin	6	27	5	med
English mustard	7	1 teaspoon	trace	trace	trace	low
Escargots à la bourguignonne	311	6 snails	12	trace	25	low
Escarole	6	1 good handful	trace	2	trace	med
Esrom cheese	84	1 small wedge	5	trace	7	0
Evaporated milk	151	100 ml/3½ fl oz/ scant ½ cup	8	8	9	0
Evaporated milk, light	80	100 ml/3½ fl oz/ scant ½ cup	10	11	trace	0
Everton mints	21	1 mint	trace	4	trace	0
Everton toffee	20	1 toffee	trace	1	0	0
Eve's pudding	222	1 serving	3	40	6	med
Exotic fruit drink	90	1 tumbler	trace	22	trace	0

Food	kCal per portion	Portion size	Protein g	Carbs g	Fat g	Fibre
Fab ice lolly	**99**	1 lolly	1	17	3	0
Faggots	**402**	2 faggots	16	23	27	low
Fairy cakes	**105**	1 individual cake	2	22	2	low
Fajitas See *individual fillings, e.g.* Beef fajitas						
Falafels	**140**	2 falafels	5	11	9	high
Fanta orange	**85**	1 tumbler	0	22	0	0
Fanta orange, diet	**6**	1 tumbler	0	0	0	0
Farfalle (pasta shapes), dried, boiled	**198**	1 serving	7	42	1	med
Farfalle, fresh, boiled	**235**	1 serving	9	45	2	med
Farmhouse loaf	**74**	1 medium slice	3	15	1	low
Farmhouse vegetable soup, canned	**90**	2 ladlefuls	4	16	1	med
Farmhouse vegetable soup, packet	**119**	2 ladlefuls	4	25	1	high
Feast ice lolly	**313**	1 lolly	3	23	13	low
Fennel	**27**	1 head	2	4	3	med
Fennel, au gratin	**145**	1 serving	7	8	10	med
Fennel, steamed or boiled	**11**	½ head	1	1	trace	med
Feta cheese	**62**	1 small chunk	4	trace	5	0
Feta cheese, with olives	**19**	1 piece of each	1	trace	2	low
Fettuccine (pasta ribbons), dried, boiled	**239**	1 serving	8	51	2	med
Fettuccine, fresh, boiled	**301**	1 serving	11	57	2	med

Food	kCal per portion	Portion size	Protein g	Carbs g	Fat g	Fibre
Fibre 1, dry	66	25 g/1 oz/½ cup	3	13	1	high
Fibre 1, with semi-skimmed milk	166	5 heaped tbsp	9	26	3	high
Fibre 1, with skimmed milk	150	5 heaped tbsp	9	26	1	high
Fig roll biscuit (cookie)	61	1 roll	1	11	2	med
Figgy duff	581	1 serving	9	80	28	high
Figs	24	1 fig	1	5	trace	high
Figs, canned in syrup	88	3 heaped tbsp	trace	25	trace	high
Figs, dried, ready-to-eat	45	1 fig	1	11	trace	high
Figs, dried, stewed	103	3 heaped tbsp	3	29	1	high
Figs, dried, stewed with sugar	143	3 heaped tbsp	3	34	1	high
Figs, with parma ham	87	1 fig plus 2 slices of ham	9	11	2	high
Filberts See Hazelnuts						
Filet-o-fish	389	1 portion	17	41	18	med
Fillet steak See Steak, fillet						
Fingers, milk chocolate	38	1 biscuit (cookie)	trace	6	1	low
Finger rolls	107	1 roll	4	21	2	low
Finnan haddie	148	1 fish	34	0	1	0
Fish and chips, deep-fried, chip-shop-style	891	1 serving	54	68	46	high
Fish cakes, salmon, fried (sautéed)	213	1 cake	8	15	11	low

Food	kCal per portion	Portion size	Protein g	Carbs g	Fat g	Fibre
Fish cakes, salmon, grilled (broiled)	**192**	1 cake	10	17	7	low
Fish cakes, white fish, fried	**188**	1 cake	9	15	10	low
Fish cakes, white fish, grilled	**169**	1 cake	11	17	6	low
Fish chowder	**285**	2 ladlefuls	44	60	10	med
Fish fingers, fried (sautéed)	**47**	1 finger	3	3	3	low
Fish fingers, grilled (broiled)	**43**	1 finger	3	4	2	low
Fish goujons	**304**	6 goujons	37	6	14	low
Fish kebabs	**95**	1 kebab	21	0	1	0
Fish mornay	**239**	1 serving	11	13	21	low
Fish mousse	**180**	1 serving	10	6	15	low
Fish paste	**25**	1 tbsp	2	trace	1	low
Fish pie, topped with pastry (paste)	**384**	1 serving	14	27	25	low
Fish pie, topped with potato	**315**	1 serving	24	37	9	med
Fish soup	**159**	2 ladlefuls	16	21	2	med
Fish stew	**330**	1 serving	30	43	5	med
Fish sticks	**76**	1 stick	4	7	3	0
Flageolet beans, canned, drained	**98**	3 heaped tbsp	7	21	1	high
Flageolet beans, dried, soaked and cooked	**104**	3 heaped tbsp	8	23	1	high

Food	kCal per portion	Portion size	Protein g	Carbs g	Fat g	Fibre
Flake chocolate bar	180	1 standard bar	3	19	10	0
Flan, fruit, any flavour	222	1 slice	3	40	6	low
Flapjack	417	1 piece	6	48	23	high
Florida cocktail	56	1 serving	trace	10	trace	low
Flounder, fried (sautéed)	378	1 small fish	28	16	23	low
Flounder, grilled (broiled)	175	1 small fish	35	0	2	0
Focaccia bread	139	1 medium slice	3	30	1	med
Fois gras	158	1 serving	6	trace	14	0
Fondant creams	25	1 sweet (candy)	trace	7	0	0
Fondant icing (frosting)	100	25 g/1 oz	0	25	0	0
Fondue, cheese	492	1 serving	30	8	29	0
Fondue, cheese, with French bread	762	1 serving plus 10 cubes of bread	40	62	31	med
Fontina cheese	110	1 small wedge	7	trace	9	0
Forcemeat balls	115	2 balls	3	10	7	low
Four cheese pizza	334	1 slice	13	36	17	med
Four cheese pasta sauce	500	¼ jar	17	76	13	med
Four seasons pizza	342	1 slice	12	32	16	med
Framboise liqueur	65	1 single measure	trace	7	0	0
Frankfurter	186	1 frankfurter	9	2	15	low
Frankfurter, canned	82	1 frankfurter	3	1	7	low
French (green) beans, canned, drained	22	3 heaped tbsp	1	4	trace	med

Food	kCal per portion	Portion size	Protein g	Carbs g	Fat g	Fibre
French beans, steamed or boiled	**25**	3 heaped tbsp	2	5	trace	high
French dressing	**97**	1 tbsp	trace	0	17	0
French dressing, low-calorie	**5**	1 tbsp	trace	1	trace	0
French fancies, fondant-iced (frosted)	**150**	1 cake	1	25	5	low
French fries, thin, from burger outlets See also Chips	**206**	1 serving	3	28	9	med
French mustard	**7**	1 tsp	trace	1	trace	low
French onion soup, canned	**48**	2 ladlefuls	2	11	trace	low
French onion soup, home-made	**94**	2 ladlefuls	2	8	6	low
French onion soup, packet	**104**	2 ladlefuls	2	20	1	low
French onion soup, with cheese croûtes	**226**	2 ladlefuls plus 1 croûte	9	21	8	low
French stick	**135**	1 thick slice	5	27	1	low
French toast	**213**	1 slice	6	17	18	low
Fried (sautéed) bread	**181**	1 slice	3	17	11	low
Fried (sautéed) egg sandwiches	**406**	1 round	13	34	25	med
Fried rice See Rice, Egg fried rice and Special fried rice						
Fries See Chips						
Frisée See Curly endive						

Food	kCal per portion	Portion size	Protein g	Carbs g	Fat g	Fibre
Frito misto	338	1 serving	24	43	11	low
Frittata	328	2 eggs	16	17	22	med
Frogs' legs, fried (sautéed)	178	2 legs	22	0	10	low
Fromage blanc	24	1 heaped tbsp	2	trace	trace	0
Fromage frais	113	1 individual pot	7	6	7	0
Fromage frais, flavoured	131	1 individual pot	7	14	6	low
Fromage frais, low-fat	58	1 individual pot	8	7	trace	low
Fromage frais, low-fat, flavoured	58	1 individual pot	8	7	trace	low
Frosted shreddies, dry	91	25 g/1 oz/½ cup	2	20	trace	high
Frosted shreddies, with semi-skimmed milk	224	5 heaped tbsp	7	43	3	high
Frosted shreddies, with skimmed milk	208	5 heaped tbsp	7	43	1	high
Frosted wheats, dry	80	25 g/1 oz/½ cup	2	17	trace	high
Frosted wheats, with semi-skimmed milk	185	5 heaped tbsp	8	34	3	high
Frosted wheats, with skimmed milk	169	5 heaped tbsp	8	34	1	high
Frosties, dry	95	25 g/1 oz/½ cup	1	22	trace	low
Frosties, with semi-skimmed milk	209	5 heaped tbsp	6	41	2	low
Frosties, with skimmed milk	193	5 heaped tbsp	6	41	trace	low
Frosties cereal and milk bar	121	1 bar	3	18	4	low

Food	kCal per portion	Portion size	Protein g	Carbs g	Fat g	Fibre
Frosting *See* Icing						
Fruit cake, light	**354**	1 slice	5	58	13	med
Fruit cake, rich *See also* Christmas cake	**341**	1 slice	4	60	11	med
Fruit chewy sweets (candies)	**185**	1 tube	trace	38	4	0
Fruit cobbler	**255**	1 serving	4	46	7	med
Fruit cocktail, canned in natural juice	**57**	3 heaped tbsp	trace	15	trace	low
Fruit cocktail, canned in syrup	**77**	3 heaped tbsp	trace	20	trace	low
Fruit corner yoghurt dessert	**219**	1 ind carton	6	26	7	low
Fruit flan, made with pastry (paste)	**153**	1 slice	2	24	6	low
Fruit flan, made with sponge	**222**	1 slice	3	40	1	low
Fruit gums	**134**	1 tube	2	32	0	0
Fruit 'n' fibre, dry	**87**	25 g/1 oz/½ cup	2	17	1	high
Fruit 'n' fibre, with semi-skimmed milk	**197**	5 heaped tbsp	8	34	4	high
Fruit 'n' fibre, with skimmed milk	**181**	5 heaped tbsp	8	34	2	high
Fruit pastilles	**147**	1 tube	2	35	0	0
Fruit pie	**241**	1 individual pie	2	39	8	med
Fruit punch	**59**	1 wine glass	0	15	0	low
Fruit salad, canned in natural juice	**29**	3 heaped tbsp	trace	7	trace	low

Food	kCal per portion	Portion size	Protein g	Carbs g	Fat g	Fibre
Fruit salad, canned in syrup	57	3 heaped tbsp	trace	15	trace	low
Fruit salad, dried	145	3 heaped tbsp	3	40	trace	high
Fruit salad, dried, stewed	83	3 heaped tbsp	1	26	trace	high
Fruit salad, dried, stewed with sugar	94	3 heaped tbsp	1	29	trace	high
Fruit salad, fresh, in pure juice	27	3 heaped tbsp	1	7	trace	med
Fruit salad, fresh, in syrup	55	3 heaped tbsp	1	14	trace	med
Fruit salad, tropical	47	3 heaped tbsp	1	9	0	med
Fruit scone (biscuit)	158	1 scone	4	26	5	med
Fruit scone, with butter	232	1 scone	4	26	13	med
Fruit scone, with low-fat spread	197	1 scone	5	26	9	med
Fruit shortcake	52	1 biscuit (cookie)	1	7	2	low
Fruit squash See individual flavours, e.g. Orange squash						
Fruitful shredded wheat, dry	88	25 g/1 oz/½ cup	2	17	1	high
Fruitful shredded wheat, with semi-skimmed milk	202	3 heaped tbsp	8	34	4	high
Fruitful shredded wheat, with skimmed milk	186	3 heaped tbsp	8	34	2	high
Fruitibix, dry	88	25 g/1 oz/½ cup	2	18	1	high
Fruitibix, with semi-skimmed milk	200	3 heaped tbsp	8	34	3	high

Food	kCal per portion	Portion size	Protein g	Carbs g	Fat g	Fibre
Fruitibix, with skimmed milk	**184**	3 heaped tbsp	8	34	1	high
Fudge *See also individual flavours, e.g. Chocolate fudge*	77	1 square	trace	14	2	0
Fudge brownie	**394**	1 brownie	5	62	20	low
Ful medames beans, dried, soaked and cooked	116	3 heaped tbsp	9	20	1	high
Fusilli (pasta spirals), dried, boiled	**239**	1 serving	8	51	2	med
Fusilli, fresh, boiled	**301**	1 serving	11	57	2	med

Food	kCal per portion	Portion size	Protein g	Carbs g	Fat g	Fibre
Gaelic coffee	**218**	1 wine glass	1	7	14	0
Gala pie	**564**	1 slice	15	37	68	med
Galaxy chocolate bar, all flavours	**250** (avge)	1 standard bar	4	27	14	0
Galaxy cake bar	**178**	1 cake bar	2	20	10	low
Galaxy cake bar, caramel	**148**	1 cake bar	2	20	7	low
Galaxy double nut and raisin bar	**246**	1 standard bar	4	26	14	0
Galaxy ice cream	**302**	1 ice cream bar	4	28	19	0
Galaxy muffin	**356**	1 muffin	5	42	18	low
Game chips	**273**	10 chips	3	25	19	med
Game pie	**606**	1 serving	21	49	35	med
Game soup, canned	**88**	2 ladlefuls	5	10	4	low
Gammon, honey-roast	**174**	2 thick slices	25	4	6	0
Gammon, lean, boiled	**167**	2 thick slices	29	0	5	0
Gammon, rasher (slice), fried (sautéed)	**171**	1 rasher	22	0	9	0
Gammon, rasher, grilled (broiled)	**141**	1 rasher	22	0	8	0
Gammon, steak, grilled	**301**	1 medium steak	54	0	9	0
Gammon with pineapple	**324**	1 medium steak plus 1 pineapple slice	54	6	9	med
Gammon and egg	**403**	1 medium steak plus 1 egg	62	trace	17	0
Garbanzos See Chick peas						

Food	kCal per portion	Portion size	Protein g	Carbs g	Fat g	Fibre
Garibaldi biscuits (cookies)	**41**	1 biscuit	trace	7	1	low
Garlic	**5**	1 clove	trace	1	trace	low
Garlic and herb soft cheese	**77**	1 good spoonful	2	1	7	low
Garlic bread	**73**	1 small slice	1	7	4	low
Garlic butter	**112**	1 tbsp	trace	trace	12	low
Garlic chicken	**316**	1 breast	40	3	16	low
Garlic mayonnaise	**237**	2 tbsp	trace	trace	23	0
Garlic sausage	**12**	1 slice	1	trace	1	low
Gazpacho	**136**	2 ladlefuls	3	trace	7	med
Genoa cake	**383**	1 slice	5	56	16	med
German smoked cheese	**60**	1 small wedge	4	trace	3	0
Ghee	**224**	25 g/1 oz/2 tbsp	trace	trace	25	0
Gherkins (cornichons)	**4**	1 gherkin	trace	1	trace	low
Gin	**55**	1 single measure	trace	trace	0	0
Gin and dry martini	**114**	1 cocktail	trace	3	trace	0
Gin and lime	**111**	1 single measure	trace	15	0	0
Gin and orange	**108**	1 single measure	trace	7	0	0
Gin and sweet martini	**130**	1 cocktail	trace	8	0	0
Gin and tonic	**76**	1 single measure plus 1 mixer	trace	5	0	0
Gin and tonic, low-calorie	**56**	1 single measure plus 1 mixer	trace	trace	trace	0
Ginger, chocolate	**30**	1 piece	trace	7	trace	low

Food	kCal per portion	Portion size	Protein g	Carbs g	Fat g	Fibre
Ginger, crystallised	30	1 piece	trace	4	0	low
Ginger, stem, in syrup	30	1 piece	trace	2	trace	low
Ginger ale, american	44	1 tumbler	0	10	0	0
Ginger ale, dry	32	1 tumbler	0	8	0	0
Ginger ale, low-calorie	1	1 tumbler	trace	trace	trace	0
Ginger beer	98	1 tumbler	0	24	0	0
Ginger cake	388	1 slice	3	60	15	med
Ginger cake bar	128	1 cake bar	1	22	4	low
Ginger ice cream	89	1 scoop	2	11	4	low
Ginger nuts	56	1 biscuit (cookie)	1	9	2	low
Ginger nuts, milk or plain (semi-sweet) chocolate	70	1 biscuit	1	10	3	low
Ginger snaps	37	1 biscuit (cookie)	trace	6	1	low
Ginger wine	200	1 double measure	trace	16	0	0
Gingerbread	180	1 slice	2	28	7	low
Gingerbread men	249	1 man	4	34	11	low
Gipsy creams	64	1 biscuit (cookie)	1	8	3	low
Gjetost cheese	132	1 small wedge	3	12	8	0
Glacé (candied) cherries	13	1 cherry	trace	4	trace	low
Glacé (candied) fruits	13	1 piece	trace	4	trace	low
Glacé icing (frosting)	56	1 tbsp	0	14	0	0
Globe artichoke, whole, steamed or boiled *See also* Artichokes	70	1 medium artichoke	0	3	0	med

Food	kCal per portion	Portion size	Protein g	Carbs g	Fat g	Fibre
Globe artichoke heart, canned, drained	8	1 heart	1	1	trace	med
Glucose, powdered or liquid	48	1 tbsp	trace	13	0	0
Gnocchi	213	1 serving	3	13	12	low
Gnocchi, with butter and Parmesan	385	1 serving	9	13	29	low
Goats' cheese, hard	128	1 small wedge	9	1	10	0
Goats' cheese, soft	152	1 heaped tbsp	10	trace	12	0
Goats' milk	180	300 ml/½ pt/ 1¼ cups	9	12	10	0
Golden cutlets (smoked, whiting), poached	166	1 medium fillet	21	0	1	0
Golden grahams, dry	93	25 g/1 oz/½ cup	1	20	1	low
Golden grahams, with semi-skimmed milk	172	5 heaped tbsp	6	30	3	low
Golden grahams, with skimmed milk	156	5 heaped tbsp	6	30	1	low
Golden nuggets, dry	95	25 g/1 oz/½ cup	1	22	trace	low
Golden nuggets, with semi-skimmed milk	174	5 heaped tbsp	6	32	2	low
Golden nuggets, with skimmed milk	158	5 heaped tbsp	6	32	trace	low
Golden raisins See Sultanas						
Golden (light corn) syrup	45	1 tbsp	trace	12	0	0
Golden syrup cake bar	385	1 cake bar	4	60	14	med

Food	kCal per portion	Portion size	Protein g	Carbs g	Fat g	Fibre
Golden syrup cake bar, mini	126	1 cake bar	1	22	4	low
Goose, roast, without skin	319	3 med slices	29	0	22	0
Gooseberries	19	3 heaped tbsp	1	3	trace	med
Gooseberries, canned in syrup	73	3 heaped tbsp	trace	18	trace	med
Gooseberries, stewed	16	3 heaped tbsp	1	2	trace	med
Gooseberries, stewed with sugar	54	3 heaped tbsp	1	13	trace	med
Gooseberry fool	183	1 serving	3	20	9	med
Gooseberry pie	314	1 slice	4	40	16	med
Gooseberry sauce	42	1 tbsp	trace	trace	4	med
Gorgonzola cheese	106	1 small wedge	4	trace	10	0
Gouda cheese	94	1 small wedge	6	trace	8	0
Gougère, cheese	239	1 serving	16	8	24	low
Goulash, hungarian	406	1 serving	28	16	22	med
Graham crackers See Digestive biscuits						
Grainy mustard	7	1 tsp	2	1	trace	low
Granary bread	94	1 medium slice	4	18	1	med
Grand marnier	78	1 single measure	trace	7	0	0
Granda padano cheese	113	1 small wedge	10	trace	8	0
Granola, dry	89	25 g/1 oz/¼ cup	3	17	1	high
Granola, with semi-skimmed milk	236	3 heaped tbsp	10	40	5	high

131

Food	kCal per portion	Portion size	Protein g	Carbs g	Fat g	Fibre
Granola, with skimmed milk	**226**	3 heaped tbsp	10	40	3	high
Grape juice	**92**	1 tumbler	1	23	trace	0
Grape juice, red	**92**	1 tumbler	1	23	trace	0
Grape juice, red, sparkling	**61**	1 wine glass	trace	16	0	0
Grape juice, white	**92**	1 tumbler	1	23	trace	0
Grape juice, white, sparkling	**61**	1 wine glass	trace	16	0	0
Grapefruit	**48**	1 fruit	2	12	trace	med
Grapefruit, canned in natural juice	**30**	3 heaped tbsp	1	7	trace	low
Grapefruit, canned in syrup	**60**	3 heaped tbsp	trace	15	trace	low
Grapefruit, with port	**47**	½ grapefruit	1	8	trace	med
Grapefruit, with sugar	**64**	½ grapefruit	1	16	trace	med
Grapefruit, with sugar, grilled (broiled)	**64**	½ grapefruit	1	16	trace	med
Grapefruit cocktail	**72**	1 serving	trace	18	trace	low
Grapefruit drink, sparkling	**88**	1 tumbler	0	24	0	0
Grapefruit juice	**66**	1 tumbler	1	17	trace	low
Grapefruit juice drink	**72**	1 tumbler	trace	18	trace	low
Grapenuts, dry	**86**	25 g/1 oz/½ cup	2	20	trace	med
Grapenuts, with semi-skimmed milk	**195**	3 heaped tbsp	8	26	2	med

Food	kCal per portion	Portion size	Protein g	Carbs g	Fat g	Fibre
Grapenuts, with skimmed milk	**183**	3 heaped tbsp	8	26	trace	med
Grapes, black	**60**	1 small bunch	trace	15	trace	low
Grapes, green	60	1 small bunch	trace	15	trace	low
Grappa	**79**	1 single measure	trace	6	0	0
Gravlax	**336**	1 serving	34	4	21	0
Gravy, made with giblets or meat juices	**56**	5 tbsp	4	2	4	low
Gravy, made with granules	**25**	5 tbsp	trace	2	2	low
Gravy, thin	**2**	5 tbsp	trace	trace	trace	0
Greek pastries	**322**	1 piece	5	40	17	med
Greek slow–roasted lamb *See* Kleftiko						
Greek pork stew *See* Afelia						
Greek village salad	**108**	1 serving	6	5	8	high
Greek-style yoghurt, cows'	**161**	1 individual pot	8	5	13	0
Greek-style yoghurt, sheep's	**149**	1 individual pot	6	8	10	0
Greek-style yoghurt, with honey	**158**	1 serving	6	15	9	0
Green beans *See* French (green) beans						
Green chartreuse	**78**	1 single measure	trace	7	0	0
Green salad	**14**	1 serving	1	2	trace	med

Food	kCal per portion	Portion size	Protein g	Carbs g	Fat g	Fibre
Green salad, dressed	111	1 serving	1	2	17	med
Greengage	13	1 fruit	trace	2	trace	med
Greengage pie	290	1 slice	3	39	14	med
Greengages, canned in natural juice	51	3 heaped tbsp	trace	11	trace	med
Greengages, canned in syrup	69	3 heaped tbsp	trace	16	trace	med
Greengages, stewed	37	3 heaped tbsp	1	6	trace	med
Greengages, stewed with sugar	117	3 heaped tbsp	1	19	trace	med
Grenadine syrup, undiluted	35	1 tbsp	trace	9	0	0
Griddle scones (biscuits)	44	1 scone	1	6	2	low
Grillsteak, minced (ground) beef, grilled (broiled)	185	1 steak	11	8	12	low
Grillsteak, minced lamb, grilled (broiled)	175	1 steak	14	1	13	0
Ground beef See Beef, minced						
Ground rice pudding, made with semi-skimmed milk	205	1 serving	8	40	11	low
Ground rice pudding, made with skimmed milk	186	1 serving	8	40	trace	low
Grouper, grilled (broiled)	238	1 piece of fillet	50	6	3	0
Grouse, roast	456	1 small bird	82	0	14	0
Gruyère (swiss) cheese	117	1 small wedge	8	trace	9	0

Food	kCal per portion	Portion size	Protein g	Carbs g	Fat g	Fibre
Guacamole	**408**	1 serving	1	1	45	med
Guard of honour, stuffed	**550**	2 lamb cutlets	30	10	42	low
Guava	**26**	1 medium fruit	1	5	trace	high
Guava, canned in natural juice	**48**	3 heaped tbsp	trace	11	0	high
Guava, canned in syrup	**60**	3 heaped tbsp	trace	16	0	high
Guinea fowl, roast	**480**	¼ bird	74	0	14	0
Guinness	**117**	1 small	1	6	trace	0

Food	kCal per portion	Portion size	Protein g	Carbs g	Fat g	Fibre
Haddock, fried (sautéed), in batter	**490**	1 piece of fillet	46	19	26	low
Haddock, fried, in breadcrumbs	**435**	1 piece of fillet	53	9	26	low
Haddock, poached or steamed	**171**	1 piece of fillet	40	0	1	0
Haddock, smoked, poached	**176**	1 piece of fillet	41	0	1	0
Haggis	**310**	1 serving	11	19	22	low
Hake, fried (sautéed), in batter	**497**	1 piece of fillet	49	19	26	0
Hake, poached or steamed	**164**	1 piece of fillet	42	0	7	0
Halibut, grilled (broiled)	**231**	1 piece of fillet	42	0	7	0
Halibut, poached or steamed	**229**	1 piece of fillet	42	0	7	0
Halloumi cheese	**98**	1 thick slice (⅛ block)	7	1	7	0
Halva	**265**	¼ block	7	23	16	low
Ham, boiled	**167**	2 thick slices	29	0	5	0
Ham, canned	**60**	1 medium slice	9	0	2	0
Ham, ready-sliced, no added water	**37**	1 medium slice	6	trace	1	0
Ham, roast	**174**	2 thick slices	25	4	6	low
Ham and cheese quiche	**476**	1 slice	23	24	32	low
Ham and chopped pork loaf	**35**	1 slice	2	trace	3	low

Food	kCal per portion	Portion size	Protein g	Carbs g	Fat g	Fibre
Ham and mushroom pizza, deep-pan	292	1 slice	8	35	11	med
Ham and mushroom pizza, thin-crust	242	1 slice	8	26	9	med
Ham and pineapple pizza, deep-pan	276	1 slice	8	31	11	med
Ham and pineapple pizza, thin-crust	226	1 slice	8	22	9	med
Ham and tomato quiche	479	1 slice	23	25	32	low
Ham sandwiches	341	1 round	11	34	18	med
Hamburger, retail	253	1 burger in a bun	13	33	8	med
Hamburger, home-made	437	1 thick burger in a bun	31	25	14	low
Hare, jugged	420	1 serving	30	7	30	low
Hare, roast	193	1 serving	30	0	9	0
Hare, stewed	192	1 serving	30	0	8	0
Haricot (navy) beans, canned, drained	92	3 heaped tbsp	7	17	trace	high
Haricot beans, dried, soaked and cooked	95	3 heaped tbsp	7	17	trace	high
Haricot mutton/lamb	252	1 serving	21	24	9	med
Harusami noodles	251	1 serving	2	57	trace	low
Hash browns	138	1 serving	1	16	8	med
Haslet	30	1 slice	2	2	2	low
Havarti cheese	100	1 slice	6	0	9	0

Food	kCal per portion	Portion size	Protein g	Carbs g	Fat g	Fibre
Hawaiian pizza, deep-pan	**276**	1 slice	8	31	11	med
Hawaiian pizza, thin-crust	**226**	1 slice	8	22	9	med
Hazelnut (filbert) ice cream	**91**	1 scoop	2	12	4	low
Hazelnuts, shelled	**162**	25 g/1 oz/¼ cup	3	1	16	high
Hearts, braised	**190**	1 serving	33	8	8	high
Hearts, roast, stuffed	**295**	1 serving	27	4	19	low
Hearts, stewed	**179**	1 serving	31	0	6	0
Herring, grilled (broiled)	**202**	1 medium fish	21	0	13	0
Herring, filleted, fried (sautéed), in oatmeal	**351**	1 medium fish	34	2	22	low
Herring, pickled	**39**	1 small fillet	2	1	3	0
Herring, rollmop	**180**	1 roll	12	6	12	0
Herring, soused	**180**	1 roll	12	6	12	0
Herring roes, fried (sautéed)	**244**	1 serving	21	5	16	low
Herring roes, on toast	**399**	1 serving plus 1 slice of toast	24	23	25	low
Hobnobs	**69**	1 biscuit (cookie)	1	9	3	low
Hobnobs, chocolate	**96**	1 biscuit	1	12	5	low
Hobnob creams, chocolate or vanilla	**63**	1 biscuit	1	8	3	low
Hoisin sauce	**27**	1 tbsp	trace	6	trace	low
Hollandaise sauce	**214**	3 tbsp	8	trace	25	0

Food	kCal per portion	Portion size	Protein g	Carbs g	Fat g	Fibre
Homewheat biscuits (cookies), chocolate	**87**	1 biscuit	1	11	4	low
Homewheat biscuits, chocolate, mini	**18**	1 biscuit	trace	2	1	low
Honey	**43**	1 tbsp	trace	13	0	0
Honey cake	**89**	1 slice	trace	14	0	low
Honey crispix, dry	95	25 g/1 oz/½ cup	1	21	trace	low
Honey crispix, with semi-skimmed milk	**209**	5 heaped tbsp	6	33	3	low
Honey crispix, with skimmed milk	**193**	5 heaped tbsp	6	33	1	low
Honey loops, dry	**92**	25 g/1 oz/½ cup	2	19	1	med
Honey loops, with semi-skimmed milk	**205**	5 heaped tbsp	7	37	3	med
Honey loops, with skimmed milk	**189**	5 heaped tbsp	7	37	1	med
Honey mustard	**7**	1 tsp	trace	trace	trace	0
Honey nut cheerios, dry	**93**	25 g/1 oz/½ cup	2	20	1	med
Honey nut cheerios, with semi-skimmed milk	**172**	5 heaped tbsp	6	30	3	med
Honey nut cheerios, with skimmed milk	**156**	5 heaped tbsp	6	30	1	med
Honey nut corn flakes, dry	**97**	25 g/1 oz/½ cup	2	20	1	low
Honey nut corn flakes, with semi-skimmed milk	**213**	5 heaped tbsp	7	39	3	low
Honey nut corn flakes, with skimmed milk	**197**	5 heaped tbsp	7	39	1	low

Food	kCal per portion	Portion size	Protein g	Carbs g	Fat g	Fibre
Honey nut shredded wheat, dry	95	25 g/1 oz/½ cup	3	17	2	high
Honey nut shredded wheat, with semi-skimmed milk	210	3 heaped tbsp	8	34	5	high
Honey nut shredded wheat, with skimmed milk	194	3 heaped tbsp	8	34	3	high
Honey rice krispies, dry	35	25 g/1 oz/½ cup	1	22	trace	low
Honey rice krispies, with semi-skimmed milk	209	5 heaped tbsp	6	42	2	low
Honey rice krispies, with skimmed milk	193	5 heaped tbsp	6	42	trace	low
Honeycomb	42	1 tbsp	trace	11	1	0
Honeydew melon	63	1 large wedge	1	15	trace	med
Horlicks, made with semi-skimmed milk	202	1 mug	11	32	5	low
Horlicks, made with skimmed milk	170	1 mug	11	32	1	low
Horlicks, instant, chocolate, made with water	128	1 mug	5	21	3	med
Horlicks, instant, chocolate malted, made with water	129	1 mug	3	24	2	med
Horlicks, instant, low-fat, made with water	127	1 mug	6	25	1	low
Horn of plenty mushrooms, fried (sautéed)	78	2 tbsp	1	trace	8	low

Food	kCal per portion	Portion size	Protein g	Carbs g	Fat g	Fibre
Horn of plenty mushrooms, stewed	6	2 tbsp	1	trace	trace	low
Horseradish, cream	11	1 tsp	trace	1	1	low
Horseradish, fresh, grated	24	1 tbsp	trace	1	1	low
Horseradish, relish	5	1 tsp	trace	trace	trace	low
Horseradish, sauce	8	1 tsp	trace	1	trace	low
Hot and sour soup	129	2 ladlefuls	12	8	6	low
Hot chocolate See Drinking (sweetened) chocolate						
Hot cross bun	148	1 bun	4	26	4	med
Hot cross bun, with butter	222	1 bun	4	26	12	med
Hot cross bun, with low-fat spread	187	1 bun	4	26	8	med
Hot dog	189	1 sausage plus 1 bun	7	22	9	med
Hot dog, sausage only	82	1 sausage	3	1	7	low
Hot dog, with onions	230	1 sausage plus 1 bun	4	4	10	med
Hot fudge sundae	180	1 sundae	3	30	5	0
Hummus	280	2 tbsp	10	13	22	high
Hula hoops See Potato hoops						
Hungarian goulash	406	1 serving	28	16	22	med
Huss See Rock salmon						

Food	kCal per portion	Portion size	Protein g	Carbs g	Fat g	Fibre
Ice cream, dairy, flavoured	89	1 scoop	2	11	4	low
Ice cream, dairy, vanilla	97	1 scoop	2	12	5	low
Ice cream, low-calorie, flavoured	67	1 scoop	2	8	3	low
Ice cream, low-calorie, vanilla	71	1 scoop	1	9	3	low
Ice cream, mixed, multi-flavours	91	1 scoop	2	12	4	low
Ice cream, non-dairy, flavoured	83	1 scoop	1	11	4	low
Ice cream, non-dairy, vanilla	89	1 scoop	2	11	4	low
Ice cream 99, with flake bar	175	1 cornet	5	31	13	low
Ice cream bombe	283	1 serving	4	18	17	0
Ice cream cone, double	222	2 scoops	5	34	8	low
Ice cream cone, single	131	1 scoop	3	22	4	low
Ice cream gâteau	227	1 slice	3	23	14	low
Ice lolly, any flavour	28	1 lolly	trace	7	trace	0
Ice pop, large	63	1 lolly	0	17	0	0
Ice pop, small	42	1 lolly	0	11	0	0
Ice split, any flavour	83 (avge)	1 lolly	1	13	3	0
Iceberg lettuce	2	1 good handful	trace	1	0	low
Iced coffee	133	1 tumbler	6	10	8	0
Iced coffee, with sugar	173	1 tumbler	6	15	8	0

Food	kCal per portion	Portion size	Protein g	Carbs g	Fat g	Fibre
Iced (frosted) fancies	150	1 cake	1	25	5	low
Iced gems	117	1 small bag	2	25	1	low
Iced tea, with sugar	89	1 tumbler	0	20	0	0
Icing (frosting) *See individual types and flavours, e.g.* Fondant icing, Chocolate fudge icing						
Instant whipped dessert, made with semi-skimmed milk	103	1 serving	3	14	6	low
Instant whipped dessert, made with skimmed milk	88	1 serving	3	14	3	low
Instant whipped dessert, sugar-free, made with semi-skimmed milk	103	1 serving	3	11	7	0
Instant whipped dessert, sugar-free, made with skimmed milk	88	1 serving	3	11	6	0
Irish coffee	218	1 wine glass	1	7	14	0
Irish cream liqueur	102	1 single measure	1	6	5	0
Irish stew	336	1 serving	14	25	21	med
Irn-bru	65	1 tumbler	0	21	trace	low
Irn-bru, diet	8	1 tumbler	0	2	trace	low
Isotonic drink	92	1 can/carton	trace	21	0	0
Italian pork sausage	216	1 sausage	13	1	17	0

Food	kCal per portion	Portion size	Protein g	Carbs g	Fat g	Fibre
Jacket potato See also Potato, baked	272	1 large potato	8	64	trace	high
Jaffa cake	48	1 individual cake	1	9	1	low
Jaffa cake, mini	26	1 small cake	trace	5	1	low
Jaffa cake muffin	416	1 bar	4	57	19	low
Jalousie, jam (conserve)	319	1 slice	3	33	20	low
Jalousie, mincemeat	321	1 slice	4	33	21	med
Jam (conserve), any flavour	39	1 tbsp	trace	10	0	0
Jam, any flavour, reduced-sugar	18	1 tbsp	trace	5	trace	0
Jam (jelly) roll, steamed or baked	391	1 slice	5	52	19	med
Jam ring biscuits (cookies)	60	1 biscuit	1	9	2	low
Jam sandwich cake	302	1 slice	4	64	5	low
Jam sandwich creams	74	1 biscuit (cookie)	1	9	3	low
Jam sponge cake	302	1 slice	4	64	5	low
Jam tart	130	1 individual tart	1	20	5	low
Jambalaya	468	1 serving	41	61	6	high
Japanese miso soup	78	2 ladlefuls	5	8	4	med
Jarlsberg cheese	105	1 small wedge	7	1	8	0
Jasmine rice	248	1 serving	3	56	2	low
Jellied consommé	32	2 ladlefuls	5	2	trace	0
Jellied eels	70	1 small serving	6	trace	6	0

Food	kCal per portion	Portion size	Protein g	Carbs g	Fat g	Fibre
Jello *See* Jelly						
Jelly (jello), any flavour	**91**	1 serving	2	22	0	0
Jelly, milk, made with semi-skimmed milk	**148**	1 serving	6	28	2	0
Jelly, milk, made with skimmed milk	**132**	1 serving	6	28	trace	0
Jelly, sugar-free, made up	**8**	1 serving	1	trace	trace	0
Jelly, yoghurt	**60**	1 serving	5	12	1	0
Jelly babies	**15**	1 sweet (candy)	trace	3	0	0
Jelly beans	**11**	1 bean	trace	3	0	0
Jelly roll *See* Jam roll *and* Swiss roll						
Jelly tots	**147**	1 small packet	trace	37	0	0
Jerk chicken	**256**	1 serving	32	15	8	high
Jerusalem artichokes, steamed or boiled	**41**	3 heaped tbsp	2	11	0	high
Jugged hare	**420**	1 serving	30	7	30	low
Jumbo shrimp *See* King prawn						
Junket, made with semi-skimmed milk	**120**	1 serving	4	16	4	0
Junket, made with skimmed milk	**101**	1 serving	4	16	2	0
Just right, dry	**90**	25 g/1 oz/½ cup	2	19	1	med
Just right, with semi-skimmed milk	**201**	5 heaped tbsp	7	37	3	med

Food	kCal per portion	Portion size	Protein g	Carbs g	Fat g	Fibre
Just right, with skimmed milk	**185**	5 heaped tbsp	7	37	1	med

Food	kCal per portion	Portion size	Protein g	Carbs g	Fat g	Fibre
Kalamares, fried (sautéed), in batter	**235**	1 serving	14	19	12	low
Kale, steamed or boiled	24	3 heaped tbsp	2	1	1	med
Kateifi	**322**	1 pastry	5	40	17	med
Kedgeree, made with smoked fish	**498**	1 serving	43	31	24	low
Kedgeree, made with white fish	**495**	1 serving	44	31	24	low
Kelp	**4**	2 tbsp	trace	1	trace	low
Kentucky fried chicken	**390**	2 pieces	29	10	27	low
Ketchup (catsup)	**15**	1 tbsp	trace	4	trace	low
Kettle chips, all flavours	**136** (avge)	1 good handful	1	12	9	med
Kidney beans See Red kidney beans						
Kidneys, devilled	**158**	1 serving	21	2	7	0
Kidneys, lambs', fried (sautéed)	**155**	2 kidneys	25	0	6	0
Kidneys, lambs', grilled (broiled)	**109**	2 kidneys	26	0	4	0
Kidneys, ox, stewed	**172**	1 serving	26	0	8	0
Kidneys, pigs', fried (sautéed)	**155**	1 kidney	25	0	6	0
Kidneys, pigs', stewed	**153**	1 kidney	24	0	6	0
Kidneys turbigo	**363**	1 serving	48	2	54	low

Food	kCal per portion	Portion size	Protein g	Carbs g	Fat g	Fibre
Kielbasa sausage, grilled (broiled)	81	1 slice	3	1	7	0
King cone	186	1 cone	2	29	7	low
King prawn (jumbo shrimp)	10	1 prawn	2	0	trace	0
King prawn, battered	45	1 prawn	2	3	2	low
King prawn, in garlic butter	48	1 prawn	2	trace	2	low
King prawn masala	164	1 serving	24	5	6	low
Kipper, grilled (broiled)	166	1 medium fish	21	0	9	0
Kipper, poached or jugged	166	1 medium fish	21	0	9	0
Kipper fillets, boil-in-the-bag	201	1 fillet	16	0	15	0
Kipper fillets, canned in oil, drained	140	1 fillet	11	trace	12	0
Kipper pâté	190	1 serving	8	trace	17	0
Kir	131	1 wine glass	trace	8	0	0
Kirsch	50	1 single measure	trace	trace	0	0
Kit kat chocolate bar	107	2 fingers	1	13	5	low
Kit kat chocolate bar, chunky	282	1 bar	4	33	15	low
Kiwi fruit	46	1 fruit	1	11	trace	med
Kleftiko (Greek slow-roast lamb with potatoes)	741	1 serving	67	11	49	med
Knackwurst/knockwurst	209	1 sausage	8	1	19	0

Food	kCal per portion	Portion size	Protein g	Carbs g	Fat g	Fibre
Knickerbocker glory	273	1 tall glass	8	41	10	low
Kohlrabi, steamed or boiled	36	3 heaped tbsp	1	5	0	med
Krackawheat	38	1 cracker	1	5	2	low
Krispen, all flavours	15 (avge)	1 cracker	trace	3	trace	low
Kulfi ice cream	340	1 serving	4	9	32	low
Kumquat	12	1 fruit	0	3	0	low

Food	kCal per portion	Portion size	Protein g	Carbs g	Fat g	Fibre
Ladies' fingers *See* Okra						
Lady fingers *See* Boudoir						
Lager	87	1 small	1	3	0	0
Lager, high-strength	226	1 small	1	7	0	0
Lager, low-alcohol	70	1 small	trace	4	0	0
Lamb, breast, roast	410	2 thick slices	19	0	37	0
Lamb, chop, lean, fried (sautéed)	277	1 chop	18	0	25	0
Lamb, chop, lean, grilled (broiled)	250	1 chop	18	0	23	0
Lamb, crown roast	488	2 cutlets	30	0	40	0
Lamb, cutlet, lean, fried	267	1 cutlet	15	0	22	0
Lamb, cutlet, lean, grilled	244	1 cutlet	15	0	20	0
Lamb, grillsteak, grilled	175	1 steak	14	1	13	0
Lamb, guard of honour	550	2 cutlets	30	10	42	low
Lamb, leg, roast, lean and fat	266	2 thick slices	26	0	18	0
Lamb, leg, roast, lean only	191	2 thick slices	29	0	8	0
Lamb, minced (ground), stewed	354	1 serving	39	0	22	0
Lamb, noisettes, fried	245	2 noisettes	28	0	14	0
Lamb, noisettes, grilled	222	2 noisettes	28	0	12	0
Lamb, shank, slow-roasted	465	1 shank	45	0	31	0

Food	kCal per portion	Portion size	Protein g	Carbs g	Fat g	Fibre
Lamb, shoulder, roast, lean and fat	316	3 medium slices	20	0	26	0
Lamb, shoulder, roast, lean only	196	3 medium slices	24	0	11	0
Lamb, steak, fried (sautéed)	357	1 steak	51	0	16	0
Lamb, steak, grilled (broiled)	334	1 steak	51	0	14	0
Lamb byriani	828	1 serving	22	75	51	med
Lamb curry	935	1 serving	37	10	82	med
Lamb curry, with rice	1183	1 serving	42	66	84	med
Lamb goulash	446	1 serving	28	16	26	med
Lamb kheema	656	1 serving	29	5	58	low
Lamb rogan josh	691	1 serving	51	17	41	med
Lamb stew	369	1 serving	16	30	13	med
Lamb tagine	724	1 serving	47	14	54	med
Lambrusco	70	1 wine glass	trace	2	0	0
Lamingtons	233	1 individual cake	3	36	2	med
Lancashire cheese	93	1 small wedge	58	trace	8	0
Lancashire hot-pot	342	1 serving	28	30	13	high
Langoustines	10	1 langoustine	2	0	trace	0
Langues de chat	28	1 biscuit (cookie)	trace	3	1	low
Lasagne, meat, home-made	650	1 serving	36	32	44	med
Lasagne, meat, ready-prepared	306	1 serving	15	38	11	low

Food	kCal per portion	Portion size	Protein g	Carbs g	Fat g	Fibre
Lasagne, seafood	351	1 serving	22	32	16	high
Lasagne, vegetable	424	1 serving	15	50	10	high
Lassi	124	1 tumbler	6	26	trace	low
Leek	44	1 medium leek	4	6	1	high
Leek, roast	67	1 medium leek	1	3	3	high
Leek, sliced, steamed or boiled	21	3 heaped tbsp	1	3	1	med
Leek and potato soup, canned	94	2 ladlefuls	2	8	6	low
Leek and potato soup, home-made	117	2 ladlefuls	5	15	5	med
Leek and potato soup, packet	80	2 ladlefuls	2	24	7	low
Leek vinaigrette	223	4 small leeks	1	3	23	med
Leerdammer cheese	93	1 small wedge	7	trace	8	0
Lemon	12	1 fruit	trace	2	trace	0
Lemon and lime, sparkling	78	1 tumbler	trace	19	trace	0
Lemon and lime, sparkling, low-calorie	9	1 tumbler	trace	2	trace	0
Lemon barley water, diluted	40	1 tumbler	trace	9	trace	0
Lemon cake	384	1 slice	5	54	18	low
Lemon cheesecake	273	1 serving	5	30	13	low
Lemon chicken	356	1 serving	58	3	13	0
Lemon curd	42	1 tbsp	trace	9	1	low
Lemon curd tart	150	1 individual tart	1	22	6	low

Food	kCal per portion	Portion size	Protein g	Carbs g	Fat g	Fibre
Lemon danish pastry	263	1 pastry	4	34	13	med
Lemon drop cakes	130	1 individual cake	1	20	5	low
Lemon drop sweets (candies)	20	1 sweet	0	5	0	0
Lemon juice, pure	1	1 tbsp	trace	trace	trace	low
Lemon meringue pie	362	1 slice	5	50	16	low
Lemon mousse	227	1 serving	4	38	8	low
Lemon puffs	69	1 biscuit (cookie)	1	7	4	low
Lemon sauce	43	2 tbsp	trace	10	0	0
Lemon sherbet sweets (candies)	20	1 sweet	0	5	0	0
Lemon slice	125	1 cake	1	19	5	low
Lemon sole, fried (sautéed), in breadcrumbs	342	1 medium fish	25	15	21	low
Lemon sole, grilled (broiled)	158	1 medium fish	25	0	4	0
Lemon sole, poached or steamed	128	1 medium fish	29	0	1	0
Lemon sorbet	65	1 scoop	trace	17	trace	0
Lemon soufflé	315	1 serving	6	21	41	0
Lemon sponge pudding	308	1 serving	3	50	11	low
Lemon squash, diluted	53	1 tumbler	trace	13	trace	0
Lemon squash, low-calorie, diluted	2	1 tumbler	trace	trace	0	0
Lemon tango	98	1 tumbler	trace	23	trace	0
Lemon tango, low-calorie	8	1 tumbler	trace	trace	trace	0

Food	kCal per portion	Portion size	Protein g	Carbs g	Fat g	Fibre
Lemon tea, instant	**88**	1 cup	trace	22	0	0
Lemon tea, instant, low-calorie	**5**	1 cup	trace	1	trace	0
Lemon water ice	**65**	1 scoop	trace	17	trace	0
Lemonade, home-made	**141**	1 tumbler	trace	35	trace	0
Lemonade, sparkling	**42**	1 tumbler	trace	11	0	0
Lemonade, sparkling, low-calorie	**1**	1 tumbler	0	trace	0	0
Lemonade shandy	**60**	1 tumbler	0	14	trace	low
Lentil and bacon soup, canned	**120**	2 ladlefuls	4	15	2	med
Lentil and bacon soup, home-made	**302**	2 ladlefuls	14	26	51	med
Lentil and tomato soup, canned	**108**	2 ladlefuls	6	20	trace	med
Lentil rissoles	**90**	1 rissole	7	15	3	high
Lentil soup, canned	**92**	2 ladlefuls	8	25	8	med
Lentil soup, home-made	**198**	2 ladlefuls	9	26	8	med
Lentil stew	**282**	1 serving	19	49	2	high
Lentils, green or brown, soaked and cooked	**105**	3 heaped tbsp	9	17	1	high
Lentils, red, cooked	**100**	3 heaped tbsp	8	17	trace	med
Lettuce	**2**	1 good handful	trace	1	0	low
Lettuce soup, rich, home-made	**127**	2 ladefuls	2	19	3	low
Light corn syrup See Golden syrup						

Food	kCal per portion	Portion size	Protein g	Carbs g	Fat g	Fibre
Lilt, pineapple and grapefruit	**90**	1 tumbler	0	23	0	0
Lilt, pineapple and grapefruit, diet	**8**	1 tumbler	0	0	0	0
Lima beans *See* Butter beans						
Limburger cheese	**93**	1 small wedge	6	trace	8	0
Lime	**9**	1 fruit	trace	1	0	0
Lime cordial, diluted	**36**	1 tumbler	trace	10	trace	0
Lime pickle	**23**	1 tbsp	trace	2	2	low
Lime squash, low-calorie, diluted	**2**	1 tumbler	trace	trace	0	0
Limeade	**16**	1 tumbler	trace	4	0	0
Limeade and lager	**54**	1 tumbler	trace	13	trace	0
Lincoln biscuits (cookies)	**43**	1 biscuit	trace	6	2	low
Lincolnshire sausage, grilled (broiled)	**117**	1 sausage	7	3	9	low
Ling, grilled (broiled)	**168**	1 piece of fillet	37	0	1	0
Linguine (pasta ribbons), dried, boiled	**239**	1 serving	8	51	2	med
Linguine, fresh, boiled	**301**	1 serving	11	57	2	med
Lion bar, chocolate	**145**	1 standard bar	1	20	6	low
Lion bar, ice cream	**227**	1 standard bar	3	24	13	low
Liqueur coffee	**218**	1 wine glass	1	7	14	0
Liquorice all–sorts	**29**	1 sweet (candy)	trace	7	trace	0
Liquorice caramels	**39**	1 sweet (candy)	trace	7	1	0

Food	kCal per portion	Portion size	Protein g	Carbs g	Fat g	Fibre
Liquorice sticks	5	1 stick	0	1	0	0
Liver, calves', braised	**165**	3 thin slices	22	3	7	low
Liver, calves', fried (sautéed), in seasoned flour	**254**	3 thin slices	27	7	13	0
Liver, lambs', fried (sautéed), in seasoned flour	**232**	3 thin slices	23	4	14	0
Liver, pigs', stewed	**189**	1 serving	26	4	8	0
Liver and bacon, fried (sautéed)	**498**	1 serving	43	8	46	0
Liver and onions, fried (sautéed)	**396**	1 serving	25	18	25	med
Liver casserole	**220**	1 serving	31	2	9	low
Liver pâté	**158**	1 serving	6	trace	14	0
Liver pâté, en croûte	**596**	1 slice	16	24	49	low
Liver pâté, low-fat	**131**	1 serving	7	2	10	0
Liver pâté, with toast and butter	**496**	1 serving plus 2 slices of toast	13	35	31	med
Liver sausage, sliced	**57**	1 slice	2	trace	5	0
Liver sausage, spreading	**77**	1 tbsp	3	1	7	low
Livers, chicken, fried (sautéed)	**194**	1 serving	21	3	11	0
Lobster	**126**	½ medium lobster	24	0	4	0
Lobster bisque	**108**	2 ladlefuls	13	10	4	low
Lobster mayonnaise salad	**363**	½ medium lobster	26	5	28	high

Food	kCal per portion	Portion size	Protein g	Carbs g	Fat g	Fibre
Lobster newburg	225	1 serving	20	23	5	low
Lobster salad	157	½ medium lobster	26	5	5	high
Lobster tails, fried (sautéed), in breadcrumbs	316	1 serving	12	29	18	low
Lobster thermidor	376	½ medium lobster	33	7	19	0
Lockets	165	1 tube	0	41	0	0
Loganberries	55	3 heaped tbsp	1	13	trace	med
Loganberries, stewed	50	3 heaped tbsp	trace	11	trace	med
Loganberries, stewed with sugar	80	3 heaped tbsp	trace	21	trace	med
Loquats	7	1 fruit	trace	2	trace	low
Low–fat spread	117	25 g/1 oz/2 tbsp	3	trace	12	0
Low–fat spread	39	1 small knob	1	trace	4	0
Lucozade	137	1 tumbler	trace	36	0	0
Lumachi (pasta shapes), dried, boiled	198	1 serving	7	42	1	med
Lumachi, fresh, boiled	235	1 serving	9	45	2	med
Lumpfish roe	40	1 tbsp	4	1	3	0
Lunch tongue	53	1 slice	4	trace	3	0
Luncheon meat	100	1 slice	4	1	9	0
Lychees	5	1 fruit	trace	1	trace	low
Lychees, canned in syrup	66	3 heaped tbsp	trace	18	trace	low
Lymeswold cheese	106	1 small wedge	4	trace	10	0

Food	kCal per portion	Portion size	Protein g	Carbs g	Fat g	Fibre
M&Ms, chocolate	219	1 small bag	2	31	1	0
M&Ms, peanut	231	1 small bag	5	26	12	low
Macadamia nuts	112	1 small handful	1	1	12	high
Macaroni, dried, boiled	198	1 serving	7	42	1	med
Macaroni, fresh, boiled	235	1 serving	9	45	1	med
Macaroni cheese	436	1 serving	23	46	17	med
Macaroni cheese, canned	188	1 small can	7	19	10	low
Macaroons, almond	120	1 macaroon	3	13	7	med
Macaroons, coconut	117	1 macaroon	1	16	5	med
Macedoine (mixed, diced vegetables), steamed or boiled	42	3 heaped tbsp	3	7	trace	high
Mackerel, fried (sautéed)	310	1 medium fish	35	0	19	0
Mackerel, grilled (broiled)	279	1 medium fish	38	0	15	0
Mackerel, smoked	531	1 fillet	28	0	46	0
Mackerel, smoked pâté	599	1 serving	19	0	58	0
Mackerel, soused	165	1 roll	16	6	9	0
Madeira, dry	58	1 double measure	trace	trace	0	0
Madeira, sweet	68	1 double measure	trace	trace	0	0
Madeira cake	393	1 slice	5	58	17	low
Madelaines	137	1 cake	2	16	8	low
Magnum, all flavours	300 (avge)	1 ice cream	4	27	20	0
Maids of honour	207	1 individual tart	2	35	12	low

Food	kCal per portion	Portion size	Protein g	Carbs g	Fat g	Fibre
Maître d'hôtel butter	92	1 tbsp	trace	trace	10	0
Malt loaf	80	1 slice	2	17	1	low
Maltesers	183	1 small packet	3	18	5	0
Mandarin orange	30	1 fruit	1	7	trace	med
Mandarin oranges, canned in natural juice	32	3 heaped tbsp	1	8	trace	low
Mandarin oranges, canned in syrup	52	3 heaped tbsp	trace	13	trace	low
Mangetout (snow peas)	16	3 heaped tbsp	2	2	trace	med
Mangetout, steamed or boiled	13	3 heaped tbsp	1	2	trace	med
Mangetout, stir-fried	35	3 heaped tbsp	2	2	2	med
Mango	97	1 medium fruit	1	24	trace	high
Mango, canned in syrup	77	3 heaped tbsp	trace	20	trace	high
Mango chutney	43	1 tbsp	trace	7	2	low
Mango mousse	137	1 serving	4	18	6	low
Mango sorbet	88	1 scoop	trace	24	trace	med
Mangosteen	20	1 fruit	trace	5	trace	med
Mangosteen, canned in syrup	73	3 heaped tbsp	trace	18	trace	med
Maple syrup	53	1 tbsp	0	15	0	0
Maraschino cherries	12	1 fruit	trace	3	trace	low
Maraschino liqueur	64	1 single measure	trace	8	0	0
Marble cake	371	1 slice	5	55	14	med
Marc	55	1 single measure	trace	trace	0	0

Food	kCal per portion	Portion size	Protein g	Carbs g	Fat g	Fibre
Margarine	**185**	25 g/1 oz/2 tbsp	trace	trace	20	0
Margarine	74	1 small knob	trace	trace	8	0
Margherita pizza, Italian-style	**235**	1 slice	9	25	12	med
Marie biscuits (cookies)	**35**	1 biscuit	trace	6	1	low
Marlin steak, fried (sautéed)	**294**	1 steak	44	0	14	0
Marlin steak, grilled (broiled)	**271**	1 steak	44	0	9	0
Marmalade	**39**	1 tbsp	trace	10	0	low
Marmalade, reduced-sugar	**21**	1 tbsp	trace	5	trace	0
Marmalade pudding	**340**	1 serving	6	45	16	med
Marmalade tart	**285**	1 slice	2	46	11	med
Marmite	**9**	1 tsp	2	trace	trace	0
Marrow (squash), steamed or boiled	**9**	3 heaped tbsp	trace	2	trace	low
Marrow, stuffed with meat	**306**	1 large slice	23	38	8	low
Marrowfat peas, canned	**100**	3 heaped tbsp	7	17	1	high
Marrowfat peas, soaked and boiled	**82**	3 heaped tbsp	6	18	1	high
Mars chocolate bar	**294**	1 standard bar	3	45	11	0
Mars ice cream	**209**	1 standard bar	3	22	12	0
Marsala	**79**	1 double measure	trace	6	0	0
Mascarpone cheese	**128**	1 heaped tbsp	trace	trace	14	0

Food	kCal per portion	Portion size	Protein g	Carbs g	Fat g	Fibre
Marshmallows	**15**	1 sweet (candy)	trace	4	0	0
Marshmallow chocolate tea cakes	**73**	1 cake	1	13	2	low
Martini, dry	**59**	1 double measure	trace	3	0	0
Martini, sweet	**75**	1 double measure	trace	8	0	0
Marzipan	**101**	25 g/1 oz	1	17	4	med
Matchmakers	**10**	1 stick	trace	1	trace	0
Matzos	**100**	1 cracker	3	23	trace	med
Mayonnaise	**104**	1 tbsp	trace	trace	11	0
Mayonnaise, low-calorie	**40**	1 tbsp	trace	1	4	0
Mcchicken sandwich	**375**	1 sandwich	16	39	17	high
Meat and potato pie	**330**	1 serving	24	25	19	med
Meat cobbler	**489**	1 serving	32	40	28	high
Meat paste	**35**	1 tbsp	1	2	3	low
Meat pie	**460**	1 individual pie	18	32	28	low
Meatballs, fried (sautéed)	**246**	4 meatballs	28	0	15	0
Meatballs, grilled (broiled)	**218**	4 meatballs	27	0	12	0
Meatballs in gravy, canned	**208**	½ large can	11	9	14	low
Meatballs in tomato sauce, canned	**227**	½ large can	8	33	7	med
Meatballs with spaghetti	**718**	1 serving	36	80	31	med
Meatloaf	**208**	1 thick slice	21	10	9	low

Food	kCal per portion	Portion size	Protein g	Carbs g	Fat g	Fibre
Meatloaf, with tomato sauce	**370**	2 slices	30	22	18	med
Mediterranean vegetables, roasted	**80**	1 serving	1	10	5	high
Melba toast	**53**	1 slice	2	11	trace	low
Melon See individual varieties, e.g. Cantaloupe melon						
Melon cocktail	**48**	1 serving	1	12	trace	low
Melon with parma ham	**105**	1 slice of melon plus 2 slices of ham	9	15	1	low
Melton mowbray pork pie	**677**	1 standard pie	18	45	48	med
Meringue	**95**	1 meringue	1	24	trace	0
Meringue, with cream	**162**	1 meringue	1	24	7	0
Meringue nest, with fresh fruit	**141**	1 meringue	3	32	1	med
Milk loaf	**60**	1 medium slice	2	12	1	low
Milk powder, dried (non-fat dried milk)	**52**	1 tbsp	5	8	trace	0
Milk, channel island	**234**	300 ml/½ pt/ 1¼ cups	11	14	15	0
Milk, condensed, skimmed, sweetened	**267**	100 ml/3½ fl oz/ scant ½ cup	10	60	trace	0
Milk, condensed, whole, sweetened	**333**	100 ml/3½ fl oz/ scant ½ cup	8	55	10	0
Milk, condensed, skimmed, unsweetened (evaporated)	**80**	100 ml/3½ fl oz/ scant ½ cup	10	11	trace	0

Food	kCal per portion	Portion size	Protein g	Carbs g	Fat g	Fibre
Milk, condensed, whole, unsweetened (evaporated)	**151**	100 ml/3½ fl oz/ scant ½ cup	8	8	9	0
Milk, semi-skimmed	**138**	300 ml/½ pt/1¼ cups	10	15	5	0
Milk, skimmed	**99**	300 ml/½ pt/ 1¼ cups	10	15	trace	0
Milk, whole	**198**	300 ml/½ pt/ 1¼ cups	10	14	12	0
Milk chocolate	**255**	1 standard bar	4	28	14	0
Milk classico ice lolly	**141**	1 lolly	2	9	13	0
Milk jelly (jello), made with semi-skimmed milk	**148**	1 serving	6	28	2	0
Milk jelly, made with skimmed milk	**132**	1 serving	6	28	trace	0
Milkshake, extra-thick	**238**	1 tumbler	6	42	5	low
Milkshake, made with granules and semi-skimmed milk	**138**	1 tumbler	6	23	3	low
Milkshake, made with granules and skimmed milk	**109**	1 tumbler	6	23	trace	low
Milkshake, made with syrup and semi-skimmed milk	**125**	1 tumbler	7	18	3	low
Milkshake, made with syrup and skimmed milk	**106**	1 tumbler	7	18	trace	low
Milk stick	**275**	1 lolly	3	24	18	0
Milky bar chocolate bar	**163**	1 standard bar	2	17	9	0

Food	kCal per portion	Portion size	Protein g	Carbs g	Fat g	Fibre
Milky way chocolate bar	**117**	1 standard bar	1	19	4	0
Milky way crispy rolls	131	1 roll	2	14	7	low
Millet flakes	**80**	25 g/1 oz/¼ cup	1	19	trace	med
Mince See *individual meats, e.g.* Beef, minced						
Mince pie, sweet	**244**	1 individual pie	2	39	9	low
Mincemeat	**41**	1 tbsp	trace	9	1	low
Minestrone, canned	**85**	2 ladlefuls	3	15	1	med
Minestrone, home-made	248	2 ladlefuls	10	39	7	high
Minestrone, packet	79	2 ladlefuls	1	15	2	med
Minibix with chocolate, dry	**96**	25 g/1 oz/½ cup	2	18	1	med
Minibix with chocolate, with semi-skimmed milk	212	3 heaped tbsp	7	35	4	med
Minibix with chocolate, with skimmed milk	196	3 heaped tbsp	7	35	3	med
Minstrels	**206**	1 small packet	2	29	9	0
Mint chocolate chip ice cream	**91**	1 scoop	2	12	4	low
Mint imperials	**18**	1 sweet (candy)	0	5	0	0
Mint jelly (clear conserve)	**38**	1 tbsp	trace	6	trace	0
Mint sauce	**18**	1 tbsp	trace	4	trace	0
Miso soup, Japanese	**78**	1 serving	5	8	4	med
Mississippi mud pie	**325**	1 slice	5	38	18	low

Food	kCal per portion	Portion size	Protein g	Carbs g	Fat g	Fibre
Mivi ice lolly, all flavours	**83** (avge)	1 lolly	1	13	3	0
Mixed (candied) peel	**35**	1 tbsp	trace	9	trace	low
Mixed salad	**31**	1 serving	2	5	1	high
Mixed salad, dressed	**128**	1 serving	2	5	18	high
Molasses	**38**	1 tbsp	trace	10	0	0
Monkey nuts, raw, shelled *See also* Peanuts	**85**	1 small handful	4	2	7	high
Monkfish, grilled (broiled)	**170**	1 piece of fillet	31	0	3	0
Monkfish, roasted	**216**	1 piece of fillet	31	0	7	low
Monkfish stew	**330**	1 serving	30	43	5	med
Monterey jack cheese	**106**	1 small wedge	7	trace	9	0
Morning rolls	**140**	1 roll	5	29	2	low
Mortadella	**47**	1 slice	2	trace	4	0
Moules à la crème	**372**	1 serving	21	11	21	low
Moules à la marinière	**238**	1 serving	21	11	7	low
Moussaka	**552**	1 serving	27	21	41	med
Mozzarella cheese, danish	**77**	1 thick slice (⅛ block)	6	trace	5	0
Mozzarella cheese, italian	**80**	¼ round cheese	5	1	6	0
Muesli, dry	**91**	25 g/1 oz/¼ cup	2	16	2	high
Muesli, with semi-skimmed milk	**203**	3 heaped tbsp	8	33	5	high

Food	kCal per portion	Portion size	Protein g	Carbs g	Fat g	Fibre
Muesli, with skimmed milk	189	3 heaped tbsp	8	33	3	high
Muffin, american	169	1 muffin	4	24	6	med
Muffin, english	127	1 muffin	5	25	1	med
Muffin, english, toasted, with butter	200	1 muffin	5	25	8	med
Muffin, english, toasted, with low-fat spread	166	1 muffin	6	25	5	med
Mulberries	43	3 heaped tbsp	1	10	trace	med
Mulled wine	105	1 wine glass	trace	5	0	0
Mullet, grey or red, grilled (broiled)	139	1 fillet	23	0	4	0
Mulligatawny soup, canned	137	2 ladlefuls	4	13	7	med
Multi-grain start, dry	90	25 g/1 oz/½ cup	2	20	trace	med
Multi-grain start, with semi-skimmed milk	201	5 heaped tbsp	7	38	3	med
Multi-grain start, with skimmed milk	185	5 heaped tbsp	7	38	1	med
Munchies	22	1 sweet	trace	3	1	0
Mung beans, dried, soaked and cooked	105	3 heaped tbsp	7	18	trace	high
Mung beans, sprouted	6	1 good handful	trace	1	trace	high
Mung beans, sprouted, canned	12	3 heaped tbsp	1	2	trace	high
Munster cheese	104	1 small wedge	7	trace	8	0
Muscatels, stoned (pitted)	41	1 small handful	trace	10	trace	low

Food	kCal per portion	Portion size	Protein g	Carbs g	Fat g	Fibre
Mushroom bhaji	123	1 bhaji	3	9	8	med
Mushroom ketchup	6	1 tsp	trace	trace	trace	0
Mushroom omelette	295	2 eggs	14	trace	26	low
Mushroom pâté	117	½ small tub	3	4	9	0
Mushroom pâté, home-made	191	1 serving	1	1	19	low
Mushroom and cheese quiche	353	1 slice	14	18	26	low
Mushroom ragu	311	1 serving	4	3	30	low
Mushroom risotto	341	1 serving	5	52	14	low
Mushroom pasta sauce	45	¼ jar	trace	7	10	0
Mushroom sauce, made with semi-skimmed milk	99	5 tbsp	3	8	6	low
Mushroom sauce, made with skimmed milk	89	5 tbsp	3	8	5	low
Mushroom soup, cream of, canned	106	2 ladlefuls	2	8	8	0
Mushroom soup, home-made	156	2 ladlefuls	7	14	2	low
Mushroom soup, low-fat, canned	48	2 ladlefuls	2	7	1	low
Mushroom soup, packet	118	2 ladlefuls	4	21	2	0
Mushroom soup, instant	96	1 mug	trace	13	5	0
Mushrooms *See also individual types, e.g.* Shiitake mushrooms	2	1 medium mushroom	trace	trace	trace	low

Food	kCal per portion	Portion size	Protein g	Carbs g	Fat g	Fibre
Mushrooms, breaded	**196**	1 serving	3	8	16	low
Mushrooms, button, sliced and fried (sautéed)	**78**	1 serving	1	trace	8	low
Mushrooms, large, flat, fried	**157**	2 large	2	trace	16	low
Mushrooms, stewed	**5**	3 heaped tbsp	1	trace	trace	low
Mushrooms, stuffed	**53**	1 large	2	4	2	low
Mushrooms à la grecque	**171**	1 serving	2	4	30	low
Mushy peas, canned	**69**	3 heaped tbsp	6	16	trace	high
Mussels, cooked, shelled	**3**	1 mussel	trace	trace	trace	0
Mussels, smoked, canned, drained See also Moules	96	½ small can	2	2	5	0
Mustard See individual varieties, e.g. Dijon mustard						
Mustard and cress	**2**	1 tbsp	trace	trace	trace	med
Mustard butter	**118**	1 tbsp	trace	trace	6	0
Mustard chicken	**176**	1 breast	26	3	5	0
Mustard sauce, made with semi-skimmed milk	**103**	5 tbsp	3	8	6	low
Mustard sauce, made with skimmed milk	**93**	5 tbsp	3	8	5	low
Mutton, boiled	**253**	2 thick slices	28	0	16	0
Mutton, haricot	**252**	1 serving	21	24	9	med

Food	kCal per portion	Portion size	Protein g	Carbs g	Fat g	Fibre
Mutton pie	**225**	1 individual pie	8	24	5	med
Mutton stew	**369**	1 serving	14	24	21	med

Food	kCal per portion	Portion size	Protein g	Carbs g	Fat g	Fibre
Naan bread, plain	175	1 small bread	6	29	4	med
Nachos with cheese	346	6 pieces	9	36	19	low
Napoletana pizza	247	1 slice	10	25	13	med
Napoletana sauce	61	¼ jar	2	9	2	low
Navy beans See Haricot beans						
Neapolitan ice cream	86	1 scoop	2	10	4	0
Nectarine	52	1 fruit	2	12	trace	med
Nesquick cereal, dry	98	25 g/1 oz/½ cup	1	21	1	low
Nesquick cereal, with semi-skimmed milk	179	5 heaped tbsp	5	31	3	low
Nesquick cereal, with skimmed milk	163	5 heaped tbsp	5	31	1	low
Nesquick milk shake flavouring See Milkshakes						
Neufchatel cheese	74	1 small wedge	3	1	7	0
Nice biscuits (cookies)	35	1 biscuit	trace	5	1	low
Niçoise salad	308	1 serving	21	34	11	high
Noilly prat	59	1 double measure	trace	3	0	0
Noisettes of lamb, grilled (broiled)	222	2 noisettes	28	0	12	0
Noodles, dried, boiled	239	1 serving	8	51	2	med
Noodles, fresh, boiled See also individual types, e.g. Chinese egg noodles	301	1 serving	11	57	2	med

Food	kCal per portion	Portion size	Protein g	Carbs g	Fat g	Fibre
Norwegian apple cake	**252**	1 slice	3	32	10	high
Norwegian blue cheese	**87**	1 small wedge	5	trace	7	0
Norwegian cream	**835**	1 serving	6	25	79	0
Nut brittle	**226**	1 standard bar	3	34	9	med
Nut cutlet	**139**	1 cutlet	5	5	10	med
Nut rissole	**203**	1 rissole	7	6	18	med
Nut roast	**366**	1 serving	12	13	29	high
Nutri-grain breakfast bars, all flavours	**130** (avge)	1 bar	1	24	3	med
Nuts See *individual varieties, e.g.* brazil nuts						
Nuts, mixed	**151**	25 g/1 oz/¼ cup	6	2	13	high
Nuts and raisins	**108**	1 small handful	3	7	7	high

Food	kCal per portion	Portion size	Protein g	Carbs g	Fat g	Fibre
Oat bran	51	1 tbsp	2	9	1	high
Oat bran crispbread	27	1 crispbread	1	5	trace	med
Oat bran flakes, dry	87	25 g/1 oz/½ cup	2	16	1	high
Oat bran flakes, with semi-skimmed milk	197	5 heaped tbsp	8	33	4	high
Oat bran flakes, with skimmed milk	181	5 heaped tbsp	8	33	2	high
Oat cereal, instant See Ready brek						
Oat flakes, dry	96	25 g/1 oz/½ cup	3	17	18	high
Oat flakes, with semi-skimmed milk	211	5 heaped tbsp	9	33	5	high
Oat flakes, with skimmed milk	195	5 heaped tbsp	9	33	3	high
Oat krunchies, dry	98	25 g/1 oz/½ cup	2	19	1	med
Oat krunchies, with semi-skimmed milk	214	5 heaped tbsp	6	25	3	med
Oat krunchies, with skimmed milk	198	5 heaped tbsp	6	25	1	med
Oatcakes	59	1 oatcake	1	8	2	med
Oatmeal	94	25 g/1 oz/¼ cup	3	16	2	med
Oatmeal porridge, made with semi-skimmed milk	207	1 serving	11	32	6	med
Oatmeal porridge, made with skimmed milk	191	1 serving	11	32	6	med
Oatmeal porridge, made with water	150	1 serving	4	26	4	med

Food	kCal per portion	Portion size	Protein g	Carbs g	Fat g	Fibre
Oats, rolled	100	25 g/1 oz/¼ cup	3	18	1	med
Oats, rolled, porridge, made with semi-skimmed milk	217	1 serving	9	35	6	med
Oats, rolled, porridge, made with skimmed milk	201	1 serving	9	35	4	med
Oats, rolled, porridge, made with water	160	1 serving	5	29	4	med
Octopus	164	1 serving	30	4	2	0
Octopus, marinated in olive oil	200	½ small can	12	2	16	0
Ogen melon	57	½ melon	2	13	trace	med
Oil, all types	135	1 tbsp	trace	0	15	0
Okra (ladies' fingers), steamed or boiled	28	3 heaped tbsp	2	3	1	high
Okra, stir-fried	269	3 heaped tbsp	4	4	26	high
Olives, black or green	7	1 olive	trace	trace	1	med
Olives, stuffed	4	1 olive	trace	trace	trace	med
Olives, with feta cheese	19	1 piece of each	1	trace	2	low
Omelette *See also individual fillings, e.g.* Cheese omelette	256	2 eggs	14	trace	22	0
Omelette arnold bennet	373	2 eggs	25	trace	29	0
Onion	36	1 medium onion	1	8	trace	med
Onion, fried (sautéed)	82	2 tbsp	1	7	5	med
Onion, pickled	4	1 onion	trace	1	trace	low

Food	kCal per portion	Portion size	Protein g	Carbs g	Fat g	Fibre
Onion, spring (scallion)	3	1 onion	trace	trace	trace	low
Onion, stuffed	190	1 large onion	13	19	8	high
Onion bhaji	123	1 bhaji	3	9	8	med
Onion dip	27	2 tbsp	4	1	1	0
Onion pakoras	148	1 pakora	3	9	11	med
Onion rings, deep-fried in batter or breadcrumbs	97	5 rings	1	9	6	low
Onion sauce, made with semi-skimmed milk	64	5 tbsp	2	6	4	low
Onion sauce, made with skimmed milk	55	5 tbsp	2	6	3	low
Onion soup, cream of, canned	88	2 ladlefuls	1	8	6	low
Onion soup, french, home-made	94	2 ladlefuls	2	8	6	low
Onion soup, french, packet	104	2 ladlefuls	2	20	1	low
Onion soup, french, with cheese croûte	226	2 ladlefuls plus 1 croûte	9	21	8	low
Onion soup, white, home-made	121	2 ladlefuls	6	12	3	low
Onion soup, white, packet	77	2 ladlefuls	trace	4	trace	low
Onions in white sauce	36	3 heaped tbsp	1	6	1	high
Orange	57	1 fruit	6	13	1	med
Orange and pineapple pure fruit juice	84	1 tumbler	1	22	trace	low

Food	kCal per portion	Portion size	Protein g	Carbs g	Fat g	Fibre
Orange and pineapple squash, diluted	**96**	1 tumbler	trace	22	trace	0
Orange and pineapple squash, low-calorie, diluted	**22**	1 tumbler	trace	5	trace	0
Orange barley water, diluted	**40**	1 tumbler	trace	10	trace	0
Orange cake	**290**	1 slice	2	32	17	low
Orange curd	**42**	1 tbsp	trace	9	1	low
Orange ice lolly	**78**	1 lolly	trace	19	0	0
Orange jelly (jello), fresh	**40**	1 serving	3	7	0	low
Orange mousse	**137**	1 serving	4	18	6	low
Orange pure fruit juice	**72**	1 tumbler	1	14	trace	low
Orange sauce	**40**	2 tbsp	trace	10	trace	0
Orange squash, diluted	**96**	1 tumbler	trace	22	trace	0
Orange squash, low-calorie, diluted	**24**	1 tumbler	0	5	trace	0
Orange tango	**92**	1 tumbler	0	25	0	0
Orange tango, low-calorie	**9**	1 tumbler	trace	2	trace	0
Orange water ice	**64**	1 scoop	trace	16	0	0
Orangeade, sparkling	**20**	1 tumbler	0	4	0	0
Oranges in caramel	**139**	1 serving	6	33	1	med
Original crunchy cereal, dry	**97**	25 g/1 oz/¼ cup	2	16	3	high

Food	kCal per portion	Portion size	Protein g	Carbs g	Fat g	Fibre
Original crunchy cereal, with semi-skimmed milk	250	3 heaped tbsp	9	37	7	high
Original crunchy cereal, with skimmed milk	234	3 heaped tbsp	9	37	5	high
Osso buco	382	1 serving	55	17	10	low
Ovaltine, made with semi-skimmed milk	197	1 mug	10	32	4	low
Ovaltine, made with skimmed milk	165	1 mug	10	32	trace	low
Ovaltine light, instant, made with water	72	1 mug	2	13	1	low
Oven chips (fries) See Chips						
Ox tongue, sliced	73	1 slice	5	0	6	0
Oxo	27	1 cube	2	4	trace	0
Oxo drink	10	1 mug	2	trace	0	0
Oxtail soup, canned	88	2 ladlefuls	5	10	3	0
Oxtail soup, packet	54	2 ladlefuls	3	8	2	0
Oxtail soup, instant	77	1 mug	1	14	2	0
Oxtail and vegetable stew	318	1 serving	38	7	15	high
Oyster mushrooms	1	1 mushroom	trace	trace	trace	low
Oyster mushrooms, fried (sautéed)	77	2 tbsp	1	trace	8	low
Oyster mushrooms, stewed	3	2 tbsp	1	trace	trace	low
Oysters	7	1 oyster	1	trace	trace	0

Food	kCal per portion	Portion size	Protein g	Carbs g	Fat g	Fibre
Oysters, fried (sautéed), in batter	**368**	6 oysters	12	40	18	low
Oysters, smoked, canned, drained	**103**	½ small can	9	trace	6	0

Food	kCal per portion	Portion size	Protein g	Carbs g	Fat g	Fibre
Paella, dried	294	1 serving	11	55	3	low
Paella, home-made	411	1 serving	40	34	11	low
Pain au chocolat	236	1 pastry	4	26	13	low
Pain au raisin	212	1 pastry	4	27	10	med
Pain perdu	213	1 slice	6	17	18	low
Pak choi/soi	19	1 head	1	2	trace	med
Pak choi/soi, steamed or boiled	12	3 heaped tbsp	1	2	trace	med
Pak choi/soi, stir-fried	36	3 heaped tbsp	1	2	2	med
Pakora	148	1 pakora	3	9	11	med
Palm hearts, canned, drained	9	1 piece	1	2	trace	low
Palmiers	83	1 piece	1	12	6	low
Pancake, buckwheat	45	1 pancake	2	6	2	low
Pancake, potato	207	1 pancake	5	22	11	med
Pancake, scotch	44	1 pancake	1	6	2	low
Pancake, wheat See also Crêpe and Drop scone	100	1 pancake	2	8	6	low
Pancake, with lemon and sugar	120	1 pancake	2	13	6	low
Pancake roll, large	217	1 large roll	7	21	12	low
Pancake roll, small	70	1 small roll	3	7	3	low
Pancetta, diced, fried (sautéed)	248	2 tbsp	11	0	22	0
Panna cotta	328	1 serving	2	38	17	low

Food	kCal per portion	Portion size	Protein g	Carbs g	Fat g	Fibre
Pappardelle (pasta ribbons), dried, boiled	**239**	1 serving	8	51	2	med
Pappardelle, fresh, boiled	**301**	1 serving	11	57	2	med
Papaya	**118**	1 fruit	2	30	trace	high
Papaya, canned in natural juice	**65**	3 heaped tbsp	trace	17	trace	low
Paratha	**450**	1 paratha	12	62	20	high
Parkin	**185**	1 piece	2	29	7	low
Parma ham	**21**	1 slice	4	0	1	0
Parma ham, with figs	87	1 fig plus 2 slices of ham	9	11	2	med
Parma ham, with melon	**105**	1 slice of melon plus 2 slices of ham	9	15	1	low
Parmesan cheese	**113**	1 small chunk	10	trace	8	0
Parmesan cheese, grated	**68**	1 tbsp	6	trace	5	0
Parsley sauce, made with semi-skimmed milk	**99**	5 tbsp	3	8	6	low
Parsley sauce, made with skimmed milk	**89**	5 tbsp	3	8	5	low
Parsnips	**112**	1 medium parsnip	3	22	2	high
Parsnips, roasted	**156**	4 pieces	3	22	6	high
Parsnips, steamed or boiled	**66**	1 serving	2	13	1	high
Partridge, roast	**212**	½ small bird	37	0	7	0
Passata (sieved tomatoes)	**29**	5 tbsp	1	6	trace	0

Food	kCal per portion	Portion size	Protein g	Carbs g	Fat g	Fibre
Passion fruit	17	1 fruit	trace	4	trace	med
Passion fruit ice cream	83	1 scoop	1	11	3	0
Pasta salad	197	1 serving	5	28	8	high
Pasta sauce, traditional, ready-made *See also individual flavours, e.g. Tomato and herb*	58	¼ jar	3	8	2	0
Pasta, shapes, dried, boiled	198	1 serving	7	42	1	med
Pasta shapes, fresh, boiled	235	1 serving	9	45	2	med
Pasta shapes, wholemeal, dried, boiled	218	1 serving	10	44	2	high
Pasta strands, all sizes, dried, boiled	239	1 serving	8	51	2	med
Pasta strands, fresh, boiled	301	1 serving	11	57	2	med
Pasta strands, wholemeal, dried, boiled	259	1 serving	31	152	6	high
Pastis	61	1 single measure	trace	trace	0	0
Pastrami	99	1 slice	5	1	8	0
Pastrami, on rye bread	154	1 slice of each	7	12	8	med
Pâté, with toast and butter	496	1 serving plus 2 slices of toast	13	35	31	med
Pavlova, topped with cream and fruit	320	1 serving	5	45	14	med
Paw paw	118	1 fruit	2	30	trace	high

Food	kCal per portion	Portion size	Protein g	Carbs g	Fat g	Fibre
Pea and ham soup, canned	**150**	2 ladlefuls	6	19	6	high
Pea and ham soup, packet	**150**	2 ladlefuls	3	18	7	med
Pea soup, canned	**188**	2 ladlefuls	10	30	6	med
Pea soup, instant	**95**	1 mug	2	16	2	med
Peach	**42**	1 peach	1	11	trace	med
Peach and apple pure fruit juice	**84**	1 tumbler	1	20	trace	low
Peach melba	**169**	1 serving	3	28	5	med
Peach pie	**261**	1 slice	2	38	12	low
Peach chutney	**24**	1 tbsp	trace	6	trace	low
Peach squash, diluted	**96**	1 tumbler	trace	22	trace	0
Peach squash, low-calorie, diluted	**24**	1 tumbler	0	5	trace	0
Peaches, dried	**31**	1 piece	trace	8	trace	high
Peaches, dried, stewed with sugar	**103**	3 heaped tbsp	1	27	trace	high
Peaches, dried, stewed	**77**	3 heaped tbsp	1	20	trace	high
Peaches, sliced, canned in natural juice	**39**	3 heaped tbsp	1	10	trace	low
Peaches, sliced, canned in syrup	**55**	3 heaped tbsp	trace	14	trace	low
Peaches, whole, poached in natural juice	**80**	1 peach	1	16	trace	med
Peaches, whole, poached in syrup	**101**	1 peach	1	16	trace	med

Food	kCal per portion	Portion size	Protein g	Carbs g	Fat g	Fibre
Peaches, whole, poached in wine	136	1 peach	1	17	trace	med
Peanut brittle	226	1 standard bar	3	34	9	med
Peanut butter	93	1 tbsp	3	2	8	high
Peanut butter and chocolate spread	89	1 tbsp	2	5	7	med
Peanut cookies	116	1 cookie	2	13	6	high
Peanut sauce	220	5 tbsp	8	8	18	med
Peanuts, dry-roasted	88	1 small handful	4	1	7	med
Peanuts, raw, shelled	141	25 g/1 oz/¼ cup	6	3	11	med
Peanuts, roasted, salted	90	1 small handful	4	1	8	med
Peanuts and raisins	70	1 small handful	3	5	5	med
Pear	45	1 fruit, unpeeled	trace	11	trace	high
Pear and apple pure fruit juice	78	1 tumbler	0	20	0	0
Pear condé	356	1 serving	4	51	15	med
Pear drops	16	1 sweet (candy)	0	4	0	0
Pear melba	179	1 serving	2	32	5	low
Pearl barley, cooked	101	1 serving	2	39	0	low
Pears, canned in natural juice	70	2 halves	trace	17	trace	med
Pears, canned in syrup	100	2 halves	trace	25	trace	med
Pears, dried	47	1 piece	trace	12	trace	high
Pears, dried, stewed	127	3 heaped tbsp	1	34	trace	high
Pears, dried, stewed with sugar	140	3 heaped tbsp	1	37	trace	high

Food	kCal per portion	Portion size	Protein g	Carbs g	Fat g	Fibre
Pears, poached in wine	139	1 pear	1	7	trace	med
Pears with chocolate sauce	348	1 serving	3	87	2	high
Peas, dried, soaked and boiled	109	3 heaped tbsp	7	20	1	high
Peas, fresh, shelled	83	3 heaped tbsp	7	11	1	high
Peas, fresh, shelled, cooked	79	3 heaped tbsp	7	10	2	high
Peas, frozen, cooked	69	3 heaped tbsp	6	10	1	high
Peas, garden, canned, drained	80	3 heaped tbsp	5	13	1	high
Peas, marrowfat, canned, drained	100	3 heaped tbsp	7	17	1	high
Peas, marrowfat, soaked and cooked	82	3 heaped tbsp	6	18	1	high
Peas, mushy, canned	81	3 heaped tbsp	6	14	1	med
Peas, processed, canned, drained	99	3 heaped tbsp	7	17	1	high
Peas, split, soaked and boiled	262	3 heaped tbsp	10	20	16	high
Peas, sugar snap	57	10 pods	5	8	1	high
Peas, sugar snap, steamed or boiled	52	3 heaped tbsp	5	5	1	high
Pease pudding	109	3 heaped tbsp	7	20	1	high
Pecan nuts, shelled	196	25 g/1 oz/¼ cup	3	2	20	high
Pecan pie	502	1 slice	6	64	27	med
Pecorino cheese	113	1 small chunk	10	trace	8	0

Food	kCal per portion	Portion size	Protein g	Carbs g	Fat g	Fibre
Peking duck with pancakes	665	1 portion with 6 small pancakes	39	32	42	high
Penne rigate (pasta shapes), dried, boiled	198	1 serving	7	42	1	med
Penne rigate, fresh, boiled	235	1 serving	9	45	2	med
Penguin chocolate bars, all flavours	135 (avge)	1 standard bar	1	17	7	low
Peperami	132	1 stick	5	trace	12	low
Peppermint cordial, diluted	36	1 tumbler	0	10	trace	0
Peppermints	18	1 mint	0	5	0	0
Peperoni	27	1 slice	1	trace	2	0
Peperoni pizza	255	1 slice	14	28	10	low
Pepper (bell), green	22	1 pepper	1	4	trace	med
Pepper, green, roasted	45	1 pepper	1	4	5	med
Pepper, green, stewed	27	1 pepper	1	4	1	med
Pepper, orange/yellow	35	1 pepper	1	7	trace	med
Pepper, orange/yellow, roasted	58	1 pepper	1	7	5	med
Pepper, orange/yellow, stewed	39	1 pepper	2	7	1	med
Pepper, red	48	1 pepper	1	10	1	med
Pepper red, roasted	71	1 pepper	2	10	6	med
Pepper red, stewed	51	1 pepper	2	10	1	med
Pepper, stuffed with meat	266	1 pepper	23	27	8	med

Food	kCal per portion	Portion size	Protein g	Carbs g	Fat g	Fibre
Pepper, stuffed with rice	202	1 pepper	7	36	5	high
Pepsi	88	1 tumbler	0	22	0	0
Pepsi, diet	0	1 tumbler	trace	trace	0	0
Pepsi max	1	1 tumbler	trace	trace	0	0
Pernod	55	1 single measure	trace	trace	0	0
Perry, sparkling	70	1 wineglass	trace	0	2	0
Persimmon	32	1 fruit	trace	8	trace	low
Pesto sauce	64	1 tbsp	1	trace	7	low
Petit pois, cooked	49	3 heaped tbsp	7	17	1	high
Petit suisse cheese	23	1 small pot	3	1	1	0
Petits fours	23	1 sweet (candy)	trace	3	1	low
Petticoat tails shortbread	64	1 wedge	1	7	3	low
Pheasant, roast	536	¼ bird	81	0	24	0
Pheasant à la normande	675	¼ bird	91	3	46	0
Pheasant casserole	588	¼ bird	85	20	30	low
Physalis	3	1 fruit	trace	trace	trace	low
Piccalilli	13	1 tbsp	trace	3	trace	low
Pickle, sweet	20	1 tbsp	trace	5	trace	low
Pickle, tomato	24	1 tbsp	trace	6	trace	low
Pickled egg	84	1 egg	7	trace	6	0
Pickled onion, large	4	1 onion	trace	1	trace	low
Pickled onion, silverskin	2	1 onion	trace	trace	trace	low
Picnic chocolate bar	230	1 standard bar	4	29	11	med

Food	kCal per portion	Portion size	Protein g	Carbs g	Fat g	Fibre
Pigeon, roast	303	½ large or 1 small bird	37	0	18	0
Pigeon casserole	333	½ large or 1 small bird	39	8	20	low
Pigeon pie	470	1 serving	40	21	28	med
Pike, grilled (broiled)	175	1 piece of fillet	38	0	1	0
Pikelets	91	1 pikelet	3	19	trace	low
Pilaff	286	1 serving	7	45	9	med
Pilau rice	212	1 serving	4	46	2	med
Pilchards, in tomato sauce, canned	177	2 pilchards	26	3	7	low
Pimientos, canned, drained	21	1 pimiento	1	8	1	low
Pimms	146	1 tumbler	trace	11	0	0
Pina colada	252	1 cocktail	1	32	3	low
Pine nuts	172	25 g/1 oz/¼ cup	3	1	17	med
Pineapple	41	1 slice	trace	10	trace	med
Pineapple, chunks, canned in natural juice	47	3 heaped tbsp	trace	12	trace	low
Pineapple, glacé (candied)	13	1 piece	trace	4	trace	low
Pineapple, with kirsch	132	2 slices	trace	29	trace	med
Pineapple and grapefruit drink, sparkling	88	1 tumbler	trace	24	trace	0
Pineapple and grapefruit pure fruit juice	94	1 tumbler	0	24	0	low

Food	kCal per portion	Portion size	Protein g	Carbs g	Fat g	Fibre
Pineapple and grapefruit squash, diluted	**96**	1 tumbler	trace	22	trace	0
Pineapple and grapefruit squash, low-calorie, diluted	**24**	1 tumbler	0	5	trace	0
Pineapple flambé	**122**	1 slice	2	24	1	med
Pineapple pure fruit juice	**82**	1 tumbler	1	21	trace	low
Pineapple sorbet	**65**	1 scoop	trace	17	trace	0
Pineapple upside-down pudding	**367**	1 slice	4	58	14	med
Pineapple water ice	**65**	1 scoop	trace	17	trace	0
Pink champagne	**114**	1 wineglass	trace	2	0	0
Pink gin	**56**	1 cocktail	trace	0	trace	0
Pink grapefruit	**48**	1 fruit	2	12	trace	med
Pink grapefruit, with sugar	**64**	½ fruit	1	16	trace	med
Pink grapefruit, with sugar, grilled (broiled)	**64**	½ fruit	1	16	trace	med
Pinto beans, refried	**237**	1 serving	6	39	3	high
Pinto beans, soaked and boiled	**137**	3 heaped tbsp	9	24	1	high
Piperade	**260**	1 serving	10	18	17	med
Pistachio nut ice cream	**91**	1 scoop	2	12	4	low
Pistachio nuts, unshelled	**50**	1 small handful	1	1	4	high
Pitta bread, party size	**16**	1 tiny bread	1	4	trace	low

Food	kCal per portion	Portion size	Protein g	Carbs g	Fat g	Fibre
Pitta bread, white	**160**	1 bread	6	36	trace	med
Pitta bread, white, small	**80**	1 small bread	3	18	trace	low
Pitta bread, wholemeal	**137**	1 bread	4	27	1	high
Pizza, cheese and tomato, deep-pan	**300**	1 slice	15	30	14	med
Pizza, cheese and tomato, thin-crust *See also other flavours, e.g.* Ham and mushroom pizza	**235**	1 slice	9	25	12	med
Plaice, grilled (broiled)	**202**	1 medium fish	23	0	7	0
Plaice, fillet, fried (sautéed), in batter	**488**	1 fillet	28	24	31	low
Plaice, fillet, fried (sautéed), in breadcrumbs,	**399**	1 fillet	31	15	24	low
Plaice, fillet, steamed or poached	**162**	1 fillet	33	0	3	0
Plantain, boiled or steamed	**112**	½ plantain	1	28	trace	med
Plantain, fried (sautéed)	**267**	½ plantain	1	47	9	med
Ploughman's lunch	**650**	1 serving	22	54	36	med
Plum, large	**30**	1 fruit	trace	7	trace	med
Plum, small	**11**	1 fruit	trace	2	trace	med
Plum crumble	**298**	1 serving	3	51	10	med
Plum fool	**227**	1 serving	5	36	8	med
Plum jam (conserve)	**39**	1 tbsp	0	10	0	low
Plum pie	**290**	1 slice	3	14	39	med

Food	kCal per portion	Portion size	Protein g	Carbs g	Fat g	Fibre
Plum pudding	291	1 serving	5	49	10	med
Plum sauce, oriental	27	1 tbsp	trace	6	trace	low
Plums, canned in syrup	59	3 heaped tbsp	trace	15	trace	low
Plums, stewed	27	3 heaped tbsp	1	6	trace	med
Plums, stewed with sugar	107	3 heaped tbsp	1	19	trace	med
Poires belle hélène	348	1 serving	3	87	2	high
Polenta (cornmeal)	214	1 serving	5	46	1	low
Polenta, with cheese	320	1 serving	9	46	14	low
Polenta, with meat sauce	431	1 serving	17	51	18	low
Pollack, baked	178	1 piece of fillet	38	0	2	0
Polish pork sausage	185	¼ ring	8	1	16	0
Polo mints	120	1 tube	0	34	trace	0
Polo mints, sugar-free	80	1 tube	0	33	0	0
Polony	70	1 slice	2	3	5	0
Pomegranate	51	1 fruit	trace	12	trace	high
Pommes dauphinoise	235	1 serving	14	12	15	med
Pompano, grilled (broiled)	186	1 piece of fillet	21	0	11	0
Pont l'évêque cheese	101	1 small wedge	6	trace	8	0
Pontefract cakes	8	1 sweet (candy)	0	2	0	0
Pop tarts, all flavours	202 (avge)	1 tart	3	36	6	med
Poppadoms, fried (sautéed)	48	1 poppadom	3	6	2	low

Food	kCal per portion	Portion size	Protein g	Carbs g	Fat g	Fibre
Poppadoms, grilled (broiled)	35	1 poppadom	3	6	trace	low
Popcorn, plain	148	25g portion	trace	16	8	med
Popcorn, sweet, buttered	122	25g portion	trace	22	4	med
Pork, chop, barbecued	210	1 chop	28	1	9	0
Pork, chop, lean, fried (sautéed)	222	1 chop	28	0	14	0
Pork, chop, lean, grilled (broiled)	199	1 chop	28	0	9	0
Pork, escalope, fried (sautéed)	185	1 escalope	31	0	7	0
Pork, loin, smoked	56	1 slice	8	0	3	0
Pork, minced (ground), lean, stewed	147	1 serving	21	0	7	0
Pork, roast, with crackling	286	2 thick slices	27	0	20	0
Pork, roast, without crackling	185	2 thick slices	31	0	7	0
Pork, sweet and sour	303	1 serving	26	31	9	med
Pork and beef sausages, thick, fried (sautéed)	115	1 sausage	5	5	8	low
Pork and beef sausages, thick, grilled (broiled)	111	1 sausage	6	5	8	low
Pork and beef sausages, thin, fried	57	1 sausage	2	2	4	low
Pork and beef sausages, thin, grilled	55	1 sausage	3	2	4	low

Food	kCal per portion	Portion size	Protein g	Carbs g	Fat g	Fibre
Pork and vegetable stir-fry	**273**	1 serving	25	18	10	high
Pork belly, grilled (broiled)	**398**	1 slice	21	0	35	0
Pork belly, pickled	**280**	1 slice	20	0	22	0
Pork chop suey	**321**	1 serving	23	34	9	med
Pork chow mein	**323**	1 serving	29	34	8	high
Pork crackling	**101**	1 finger-sized piece	trace	0	13	0
Pork kebab, marinated and grilled (broiled)	**227**	1 kebab	22	12	10	0
Pork pie	**677**	1 individual pie	18	45	49	med
Pork rillettes	**115**	2 tbsp	5	0	10	0
Pork sausages, extra-lean, fried (sautéed)	**92**	1 sausage	6	4	5	low
Pork sausages, extra-lean, grilled (broiled)	**84**	1 sausage	6	4	5	low
Pork sausages, thick, fried	**123**	1 sausage	5	4	10	low
Pork sausages, thick, grilled	**117**	1 sausage	7	5	10	low
Pork sausages, thin, fried	**61**	1 sausage	3	2	5	low
Pork sausages, thin, grilled	**58**	1 sausage	3	2	5	low
Pork spare ribs, barbecued american-style	**288**	2 ribs	25	2	16	0

Food	kCal per portion	Portion size	Protein g	Carbs g	Fat g	Fibre
Pork spare ribs, chinese-style	310	2 ribs	25	13	17	low
Pork teriyaki	133	1 serving	18	2	5	low
Porridge, instant *See* Ready brek						
Porridge, made with semi-skimmed milk	217	1 serving	9	35	6	med
Porridge, made with skimmed milk	201	1 serving	9	35	4	med
Porridge, made with water	160	1 serving	5	29	4	med
Port salut cheese	100	1 small wedge	7	trace	8	0
Port, ruby, tawny or white	78	1 double measure	trace	6	0	0
Pot au chocolat	136	1 individual pot	2	19	5	low
Pot au chocolat, with cream	270	1 individual pot	2	20	19	low
Pot noodle, all flavours	305 (avge)	1 pot	9	42	10	low
Potato, baked in jacket	272	1 large potato	8	64	trace	high
Potato, baked in jacket, with butter	346	1 large potato	8	64	8	high
Potato cake	126	1 cake	2	16	5	low
Potato chips *See* Crisps						
Potato hoops, all flavours	131 (avge)	1 small packet	1	14	8	low
Potato pancake	207	1 pancake	5	22	11	med
Potato salad, canned	176	3 heaped tbsp	2	15	10	low

Food	kCal per portion	Portion size	Protein g	Carbs g	Fat g	Fibre
Potato salad, with French dressing	**217**	3 heaped tbsp	3	27	11	med
Potato salad, with mayonnaise, home-made	**200**	3 heaped tbsp	3	17	12	med
Potato waffle, cooked	**84**	1 waffle	1	13	3	low
Potato wedges	**205**	6 wedges	10	34	4	high
Potatoes, chipped (fries), home-made	**312**	1 serving	6	50	11	high
Potatoes, creamed	**104**	1 serving	2	15	4	med
Potatoes, croquette, shallow-fried	**107**	1 croquette	2	11	6	med
Potatoes, duchesse	**82**	1 piece	2	8	2	med
Potatoes, mashed, instant	**57**	3 heaped tbsp	1	13	trace	low
Potatoes, mashed, with butter or margarine	**104**	3 heaped tbsp	2	15	4	med
Potatoes, new, boiled or steamed	**75**	3 small potatoes	1	18	trace	med
Potatoes, new, canned	**63**	3 small potatoes	1	15	trace	low
Potatoes, steamed	**72**	2 pieces	2	17	trace	med
Potatoes, roast	**149**	2 pieces	3	26	4	med
Potatoes, scalloped	**86**	1 serving	3	11	4	med
Potted cheese	**267**	1 small pot	12	1	23	0
Potted prawns (shrimp)	**358**	1 small pot	16	0	32	0
Potted shrimps	**324**	1 small pot	10	0	31	0

Food	kCal per portion	Portion size	Protein g	Carbs g	Fat g	Fibre
Poussin (cornish hen), roast, with skin	**668**	1 bird	57	0	47	0
Poussin, roast, without skin	**295**	1 bird	51	0	8	0
Poussin, spatchcocked, grilled (broiled)	**428**	1 bird	36	0	30	0
Praline ice cream	**91**	1 scoop	2	12	4	low
Prawn, king (jumbo shrimp), plain-cooked	**10**	1 prawn	2	0	trace	0
Prawn and vegetable stir-fry	**250**	**1 serving**	**20**	**30**	**5**	**med**
Prawn and avocado sandwiches	**454**	1 round	11	35	30	med
Prawn and lettuce sandwiches	**347**	1 round	10	34	18	med
Prawn byriani	**707**	1 serving	11	75	32	med
Prawn chop suey	**225**	1 serving	16	34	2	med
Prawn choux balls	**79**	1 ball	3	2	8	low
Prawn chow mein	**262**	1 serving	5	28	1	high
Prawn cocktail	**160**	1 serving	12	4	9	low
Prawn crackers	**44**	1 small handful	trace	10	1	low
Prawn curry	**220**	1 serving	8	36	5	med
Prawn fajitas	**300**	2 fajitas	15	34	13	high
Prawn jalfrezi	**465**	1 serving	26	54	9	high
Prawn mayonnaise sandwiches	**513**	1 round	10	36	27	med
Prawn risotto	**389**	1 serving	47	84	18	low

Food	kCal per portion	Portion size	Protein g	Carbs g	Fat g	Fibre
Prawn rogan josh	562	1 serving	34	17	27	med
Prawn salad	137	1 serving	26	5	2	high
Prawn salad, dressed	240	1 serving	26	5	13	high
Prawn toast	53	1 toast	2	2	4	low
Prawns (shrimp), canned, drained	80	½ small can	18	0	1	0
Prawns, cooked, peeled	53	2 tbsp	12	0	1	0
Prawns in garlic butter	284	1 serving	12	trace	24	0
Pretzel flipz	235	1 small bag	4	33	9	low
Pretzels	20	1 small handful	trace	4	trace	low
Prickly pear	42	1 fruit	1	10	trace	high
Processed cheese slice	65	1 slice	4	trace	5	0
Profiteroles with chocolate sauce	373	1 serving	6	33	24	med
Provolone cheese	99	1 small wedge	7	1	7	0
Prune juice	136	1 tumbler	1	36	trace	low
Prunes	11	1 prune	trace	3	trace	high
Prunes, canned in natural juice	79	3 heaped tbsp	1	20	trace	high
Prunes, canned in syrup	90	3 heaped tbsp	1	23	trace	high
Ptarmigan, roast	216	1 small or ½ large	38	0	8	0
Puffed wheat, dry	80	25 g/1 oz/½ cup	4	17	trace	med
Puffed wheat, with semi-skimmed milk	185	5 heaped tbsp	10	33	2	med
Puffed wheat, with skimmed milk	169	5 heaped tbsp	10	33	trace	med

Food	kCal per portion	Portion size	Protein g	Carbs g	Fat g	Fibre
Pumpernickel	93	1 slice	3	20	trace	med
Pumpkin, canned	34	3 heaped tbsp	1	8	trace	med
Pumpkin, steamed or boiled	13	3 heaped tbsp	1	2	trace	med
Pumpkin pie	316	1 slice	7	41	14	low
Pumpkin seeds	81	1 small handful	4	3	7	high
Puri	328	1 piece	7	43	25	med

Food	kCal per portion	Portion size	Protein g	Carbs g	Fat g	Fibre
Quail, roast	**205**	1 bird	37	0	6	0
Quail's eggs, cooked	**15**	1 egg	1	trace	1	0
Quality street chocolates	**37**	1 sweet (candy)	trace	5	2	0
Quark	**15**	1 tablespoon	2	trace	trace	0
Quarterpounder with cheese	**516**	1 burger in a bun	31	37	27	high
Quavers	**96**	1 small packet	trace	9	6	low
Queen cakes	**245**	1 individual cake	2	26	15	low
Queen of puddings	**341**	1 serving	11	46	13	low
Queen scallops, poached or steamed	**12**	4 scallops	2	0	trace	0
Quenelles, fish	**90**	1 ball/roll	5	3	7	0
Quesadillas	**225**	3 pieces	12	27	9	high
Quiche anglaise	**387**	1 slice	19	17	31	low
Quiche lorraine *See also individual flavours, e.g. Cheese and onion quiche*	**476**	1 slice	23	24	32	low
Quince	**17**	1 fruit	trace	4	trace	low
Quince jelly (clear conserve)	**55**	1 tbsp	trace	13	trace	0
Quinoa	**93**	25 g/1 oz/3 tbsp	3	17	1	med
Quinoa porridge, made with semi-skimmed milk	**206**	1 serving	9	34	4	med
Quinoa porridge, made with skimmed milk	**190**	1 serving	9	34	2	med

Food	kCal per portion	Portion size	Protein g	Carbs g	Fat g	Fibre
Quinoa wholegrain cereal	149	1 serving	5	28	2	med
Quorn, chunks	74	1 serving	10	2	3	high
Quorn, fillets	44	1 fillet	7	2	1	med
Quorn, fillets, in breadcrumbs	185	1 fillet	10	13	10	high
Quorn, minced (ground)	79	1 serving	13	1	3	high
Quorn, sweet and sour	149	1 serving	5	29	1	med
Quorn burger	117	1 burger	13	6	5	high
Quorn cottage pie	212	1 serving	8	32	6	med
Quorn fajitas	303	2 fajitas	14	45	7	high
Quorn sausages	115	1 sausage	13	5	5	high
Quorn southern burgers	178	1 burger	11	12	10	high
Quorn spaghetti bolognese	292	1 serving	23	38	6	high
Quorn tikka masala, with rice	540	1 serving	20	74	21	high

Food	kCal per portion	Portion size	Protein g	Carbs g	Fat g	Fibre
Rabbit and vegetable stew	404	1 serving	38	35	3	high
Radicchio	6	½ head	trace	1	trace	med
Radish	1	1 radish	trace	trace	trace	low
Radish, winter	12	1 radish	1	2	trace	low
Rainbow trout, grilled (broiled)	240	1 medium fish	34	0	10	0
Raisin bread	86	1 slice	2	15	7	low
Raisin fudge	87	1 square	trace	15	2	low
Raisin wheats, dry	80	25 g/1 oz/½ cup	2	17	trace	high
Raisin wheats, with semi-skimmed milk	185	3 heaped tbsp	8	34	3	high
Raisin wheats, with skimmed milk	169	3 heaped tbsp	8	34	1	high
Raisins, seedless	41	1 small handful	trace	10	trace	high
Raisins, stoned (pitted)	41	1 small handful	trace	11	trace	high
Rambutans	7	1 fruit	trace	2	trace	low
Rambutans, canned in syrup	82	3 heaped tbsp	1	21	trace	low
Raspberries	25	3 heaped tbsp	1	5	trace	med
Raspberries, canned in natural juice	71	3 heaped tbsp	1	17	trace	med
Raspberries, canned in syrup	88	3 heaped tbsp	1	22	trace	med
Raspberries, stewed	20	3 heaped tbsp	trace	4	trace	med
Raspberries, stewed with sugar	48	3 heaped tbsp	1	11	trace	med

Food	kCal per portion	Portion size	Protein g	Carbs g	Fat g	Fibre
Raspberry jam (conserve)	**39**	1 tbsp	trace	10	0	0
Raspberry milkshake, made with granules *See also* Milkshake	**138**	1 tumbler	6	23	3	low
Raspberry mousse	**137**	1 serving	4	18	6	low
Raspberry pavlova	**320**	1 serving	5	45	14	med
Raspberry ripple ice cream	**96**	1 scoop	4	12	4	0
Raspberry sauce	**28**	2 tbsp	trace	7	trace	med
Raspberry sorbet	**57**	1 scoop	trace	19	trace	low
Raspberry soufflé	**315**	1 serving	6	21	41	0
Raspberry tart	**271**	1 slice	3	24	18	low
Ratafia biscuits (cookies)	**21**	1 biscuit	trace	4	trace	low
Ratatouille	**191**	3 heaped tbsp	2	11	15	high
Ravioli, dried, boiled	**291**	1 serving	9	45	6	med
Ravioli, fresh, boiled	**248**	1 serving	12	32	8	med
Ravioli, in beef and tomato sauce, canned	**154**	½ large can	7	23	5	med
Ravioli, in tomato sauce, canned	**140**	½ large can	6	20	4	med
Ray *See* Skate						
Ready-to-roll icing (frosting)	**96**	25 g/1 oz	0	23	0	0
Ready brek, dry	**89**	25 g/1 oz/½ cup	3	15	2	med
Ready brek, with semi-skimmed milk	**210**	5 heaped tbsp	9	31	6	high

Food	kCal per portion	Portion size	Protein g	Carbs g	Fat g	Fibre
Ready brek, with skimmed milk	**191**	5 heaped tbsp	9	31	3	high
Ready brek, chocolate, dry	**90**	25 g/1 oz/½ cup	2	16	2	med
Ready brek, chocolate, with skimmed milk	**199**	5 heaped tbsp	9	33	3	high
Ready brek, chocolate, with semi-skimmed milk	**215**	5 heaped tbsp	9	33	5	high
Real fruit winders, all flavours	**55** (avge)	1 roll	trace	11	1	low
Red beet *See* Beetroot						
Red bull	**45**	1 can	0	11	0	0
Red kidney beans, canned, drained	**100**	3 heaped tbsp	7	18	1	high
Red kidney beans, dried, soaked and cooked	**103**	3 heaped tbsp	8	17	trace	high
Red leicester cheese	**101**	1 small wedge	6	trace	8	0
Red salmon *See* Salmon						
Red snapper, baked, stuffed	**146**	1 medium fish	19	12	2	low
Red snapper, grilled (broiled)	**218**	1 medium fish	45	0	3	0
Red windsor cheese	**100**	1 small wedge	6	trace	8	0
Red wine sauce	**63**	5 tbsp	1	9	2	0
Redcurrant jelly (clear conserve)	**55**	1 tbsp	trace	13	trace	0
Redcurrants	**28**	3 heaped tbsp	1	7	trace	high

Food	kCal per portion	Portion size	Protein g	Carbs g	Fat g	Fibre
Redcurrants, frosted	27	1 small bunch	1	7	trace	high
Refried beans	237	1 serving	6	39	3	high
Revels	173	1 small packet	2	23	6	0
Rhubarb, canned in syrup	31	3 heaped tbsp	trace	8	trace	low
Rhubarb, stewed	7	3 heaped tbsp	1	1	trace	med
Rhubarb, stewed with sugar	48	3 heaped tbsp	1	11	trace	med
Rhubarb crumble	297	1 serving	3	51	10	med
Rhubarb fool	237	1 serving	5	38	8	med
Rhubarb pie	290	1 slice	3	14	39	med
Rhubarb sauce	137	2 tbsp	1	34	trace	med
Ribena, diluted	103	1 tumbler	trace	27	0	0
Rice, long-grain, boiled	248	1 serving	5	56	2	low
Rice, brown, boiled	254	1 serving	5	58	2	med
Rice, fried (sautéed) See also Egg fried rice and Special fried rice	236	1 serving	4	45	6	med
Rice, savoury	256	1 serving	5	47	6	med
Rice and peas	247	1 serving	6	53	3	high
Rice cakes	35	1 individual cake	1	7	trace	low
Rice drink	100	1 tumbler	trace	20	trace	0
Rice, Jasmine	240	1 serving	3	56	2	low
Rice krispies, dry	92	25 g/1 oz/½ cup	1	21	trace	low
Rice krispies, with semi-skimmed milk	205	5 heaped tbsp	6	40	2	low

Food	kCal per portion	Portion size	Protein g	Carbs g	Fat g	Fibre
Rice krispies, with skimmed milk	189	5 heaped tbsp	6	40	trace	low
Rice milk	150	300 ml/½ pt/ 1¼ cups	trace	30	1	0
Rice noodles, boiled	251	1 serving	2	57	trace	low
Rice pudding, canned	323	½ large can	4	43	15	low
Rice pudding, canned, low-fat	136	½ large can	7	23	2	low
Rice pudding, made with semi-skimmed milk	150	1 serving	6	29	2	low
Rice pudding, made with skimmed milk	134	1 serving	6	29	trace	low
Rich tea biscuits (cookies)	39	1 biscuit	1	6	1	low
Ricicles, dry	90	25 g/1 oz/½ cup	1	22.2	0.2	low
Ricicles, with semi-skimmed milk	201	5 heaped tbsp	4	15	2	low
Ricicles, with skimmed milk	185	5 heaped tbsp	4	15	trace	low
Ricotta cheese, made with semi-skimmed milk	38	1 heaped tbsp	2	trace	2	0
Ricotta cheese, whole milk	42	1 heaped tbsp	2	trace	4	0
Rigatoni (pasta shapes), dried, boiled	198	1 serving	7	42	1	med
Rigatoni, fresh, boiled	235	1 serving	9	45	2	med
Ripple chocolate bar	175	1 standard bar	3	19	10	0

Food	kCal per portion	Portion size	Protein g	Carbs g	Fat g	Fibre
Risotto *See also individual flavours, e.g.* Mushroom risotto	336	1 serving	4	52	14	low
Risotto, sprinkled with cheese	449	1 serving	14	52	22	low
Risotto alla milanese	403	1 serving	7	58	18	low
Rissoles	134	1 rissole	5	8	9	low
Ritz original crackers	17	1 cracker	trace	1	1	low
Ritz cheese crackers	17	1 cracker	trace	1	1	low
Ritz cheese sandwich crackers	45	1 cracker	1	5	2	low
Riva chocolate bar	136	1 standard bar	2	14	8	low
Roasted nut cereal bar	181	1 bar	3	24	8	med
Rock cakes	176	1 individual cake	3	27	7	low
Rock salmon fried (sautéeed), in batter	580	1 fillet	30	21	44	low
Rocket (arugula)	2	1 good handful	trace	trace	trace	med
Rocky chocolate bars, all flavours	125 (avge)	1 standard bar	2	15	7	low
Roes *See* Cod roes *and* Herring roes						
Rollmop herring	180	1 roll	12	6	12	0
Rolos	269	1 tube	2	38	12	0
Romano cheese	110	1 small wedge	9	1	8	0
Root beer	135	1 tumbler	0	35	0	0
Roquefort cheese	105	1 small wedge	6	trace	9	0

Food	kCal per portion	Portion size	Protein g	Carbs g	Fat g	Fibre
Rose hip syrup, undiluted	35	1 tbsp	trace	9	0	0
Roses chocolates	39	1 sweet (candy)	trace	5	2	0
Rosti	156	1 serving	3	25	5	med
Rotelli (pasta shapes), dried, boiled	198	1 serving	7	42	1	med
Rotelli, fresh, boiled	235	1 serving	9	45	2	med
Rouille	151	1 tbsp	1	2	15	low
Roulade See individual flavours, e.g. Chocolate roulade						
Roulé, garlic and herb cheese	77	1 good spoonful	2	1	7	low
Roulé, light	28	1 good spoonful	2	1	2	0
Royal game soup	88	2 ladlefuls	5	10	4	low
Royal icing (frosting)	58	1 tbsp	trace	15	0	0
Rum, dark	55	1 single measure	trace	trace	0	0
Rum, white	55	1 single measure	trace	trace	0	0
Rum and black	123	1 single measure	trace	18	0	0
Rum and coke	94	1 single measure plus 1 mixer	trace	6	0	0
Rum and low-calorie cola	56	1 single measure plus 1 mixer	trace	trace	0	0
Rum and raisin fudge	87	1 square	trace	15	2	0
Rum and raisin ice cream	124	1 scoop	2	12	4	low
Rum and raisin sauce	145	2 tbsp	1	32	2	low

Food	kCal per portion	Portion size	Protein g	Carbs g	Fat g	Fibre
Rum baba	326	1 individual cake	4	47	10	low
Rum butter	73	1 tbsp	trace	8	4	0
Rum punch	116	1 wine glass	trace	15	trace	0
Rum sauce, made with semi-skimmed milk	50	5 tbsp	1	5	2	low
Rum sauce, made with skimmed milk	47	5 tbsp	1	5	trace	low
Rump steak See Steak, rump or sirloin						
Runner beans, steamed or boiled	18	3 heaped tbsp	1	2	trace	med
Ruote (pasta shapes), dried, boiled	198	1 serving	7	42	1	med
Ruote, fresh, boiled	235	1 serving	9	45	2	med
Russian salad	62	2 tbsp	2	5	4	high
Rutabaga See Swede						
Rye bread	55	1 medium slice	2	11	trace	med
Rye bread, light	35	1 medium slice	2	12	trace	med
Ryvita	27	1 crispbread	1	5	trace	med

Food	kCal per portion	Portion size	Protein g	Carbs g	Fat g	Fibre
Sabayon sauce	43	5 tbsp	1	4	1	0
Sag aloo	163	1 serving	5	21	9	high
Sage derby cheese	101	1 small wedge	6	trace	9	0
Sago pudding, canned	167	½ large can	4	27	7	low
Sago pudding, made with semi-skimmed milk	150	1 serving	6	29	2	low
Sago pudding, made with skimmed milk	134	1 serving	6	29	trace	low
Saint paulin cheese	100	1 small wedge	7	trace	8	0
Saithe *See* Coley						
Salad cream	52	1 tbsp	trace	2	5	0
Salad cream, reduced-calorie	29	1 tbsp	trace	1	2	0
Salade niçoise	308	1 serving	21	34	11	high
Salami, hard-cured	41	1 slice	2	trace	3	0
Salami, moist-cured	57	1 slice	3	trace	5	0
Salmon, baked, stuffed	199	1 steak	26	5	8	low
Salmon, canned, drained	155	½ small can	10	0	4	0
Salmon, grilled (broiled)	367	1 piece of fillet	39	0	25	0
Salmon, in filo pastry (paste)	495	1 portion	42	8	17	low
Salmon, poached or steamed	345	1 piece of fillet	35	0	23	0
Salmon, smoked *See also entries for* Smoked salmon	119	2 thin slices	21	0	4	0

Food	kCal per portion	Portion size	Protein g	Carbs g	Fat g	Fibre
Salmon, with hollandaise sauce	559	1 serving	43	trace	48	0
Salmon and cucumber sandwiches	378	1 round	14	35	21	med
Salmon en croûte	757	1 serving	26	46	54	low
Salmon fish cakes, fried (sautéed)	213	1 cake	8	15	11	low
Salmon fish cakes, grilled (broiled)	192	1 cake	10	17	7	low
Salmon mousse	205	1 serving	9	6	6	low
Salmon paste	33	1 tbsp	2	trace	2	0
Salmon pâté	308	1 serving	12	0	28	0
Salmon quiche	363	1 slice	17	17	25	low
Salmon salad	376	1 serving	37	5	24	high
Salmon salad, with mayonnaise	582	1 serving	37	5	47	high
Salmon sandwiches	374	1 round	14	34	21	med
Salsa, fresh chilli	18	1 tbsp	trace	4	trace	med
Salsa, fresh tomato	14	1 tbsp	trace	1	1	med
Salsify, steamed or boiled	23	3 heaped tbsp	1	9	trace	high
Saltwater crayfish See Dublin bay prawns						
Sambal	20	2 tbsp	1	4	1	med
Samosa, meat	300	1 samosa	2	9	28	low
Samosa, vegetable	236	1 samosa	1	11	21	med
Sangria	66	1 wine glass	trace	4	0	0

Food	kCal per portion	Portion size	Protein g	Carbs g	Fat g	Fibre
Sardine and tomato paste	23	1 tbsp	3	trace	1	0
Sardine pâté	238	1 serving	6	0	24	0
Sardines, canned in oil, drained	108	½ small can	12	0	7	0
Sardines, canned in tomato sauce	88	½ small can	9	trace	6	low
Sardines, canned, on toast	263	3 sardines plus 1 slice of toast	15	8	15	low
Sardines, fresh, grilled (broiled)	67	1 good-sized fish	7	0	4	0
Satsuma	23	1 fruit	trace	5	trace	med
Sauerkraut, drained	19	3 heaped tbsp	1	4	trace	med
Sausage and bacon rolls	105	1 roll	12	1	24	low
Sausage and egg mcmuffin	427	1 portion	23	25	26	med
Sausage in batter, fried (sautéed)	235	1 sausage	7	23	15	low
Sausage mcmuffin	360	1 portion	13	26	23	med
Sausage roll, cocktail	52	1 small roll	1	3	1	low
Sausage roll, jumbo	477	1 large roll	4	22	24	med
Sausage roll, puff pastry (paste)	238	1 standard roll	3	16	18	low
Sausage roll, shortcrust pastry (basic pie crust)	229	1 standard roll	4	18	16	low
Sausages See *individual meats*, e.g. Pork sausages						

Food	kCal per portion	Portion size	Protein g	Carbs g	Fat g	Fibre
Savarin	326	1 slice	4	47	10	low
Saveloy	170	1 sausage	6	6	13	low
Savoury rice, cooked	109	1 serving	3	24	0	med
Scallion See Spring onion						
Scallops, fried (sautéed), in breadcrumbs	32	1 scallop	5	1	1	low
Scallops, steamed or poached	12	1 scallop	2	0	trace	0
Scallops mornay	210	1 serving	27	18	3	low
Scaloppine, fried (sautéed), in breadcrumbs	335	1 scallopine	32	20	15	low
Scampi, fried (sautéed), in batter	360	8 pieces	16	24	16	low
Scampi, fried (sautéed), in breadcrumbs	316	8 pieces	12	29	17	low
Scampi provençal	286	1 serving	25	9	10	med
Schloer	61	1 tumbler	trace	16	0	0
Schnapps	55	1 single measure	trace	trace	0	0
Schnitzel, fried (sautéed), in breadcrumbs	335	1 schnitzel	32	20	15	low
Scone (biscuit)	181	1 scone	4	27	7	low
Scone, cheese	175	1 scone	5	21	9	low
Scone, drop (small pancake)	44	1 pancake	1	6	2	low
Scone, fruit	158	1 scone	4	26	5	low

Food	kCal per portion	Portion size	Protein g	Carbs g	Fat g	Fibre
Scone, griddle	44	1 scone	1	6	2	low
Scone, plain, with butter	255	1 scone	4	27	15	low
Scone, plain, with low-fat spread	220	1 scone	5	27	11	low
Scone, sweet	201	1 scone	4	32	7	low
Scone, sweet, with butter	275	1 scone	4	32	15	low
Scone, sweet, with low-fat spread	240	1 scone	5	32	11	low
Scone, with clotted cream and jam (conserve)	308	1 scone	4	37	16	low
Scotch broth, canned	88	2 ladlefuls	4	14	2	med
Scotch broth, home-made	156	2 ladlefuls	12	19	3	high
Scotch egg	301	1 egg	14	16	20	low
Scotch pancake	44	1 pancake	1	6	2	low
Scotch pie	225	1 individual pie	8	24	5	med
Scotch woodcock	487	1 slice	19	18	39	low
Scrambled eggs on toast	463	2 eggs plus 1 slice of toast	16	19	37	low
Sea bass, grilled (broiled)	153	1 piece of fillet	28	0	4	0
Seafood cocktail	134	1 cocktail	6	4	9	low
Seafood enchiladas	562	2 enchiladas	32	78	14	med
Seafood lasagne	351	1 serving	22	32	16	high
Seafood pasta	460	1 serving	40	62	4	high
Seafood pasta salad	261	1 serving	24	29	5	med

Food	kCal per portion	Portion size	Protein g	Carbs g	Fat g	Fibre
Seafood pizza, thin-crust	**250**	1 slice	12	25	13	med
Seafood pizza, deep-pan	**315**	1 slice	18	30	15	med
Seafood salad	**106**	1 serving	17	5	2	high
Seafood salad, with mayonnaise	**312**	1 serving	17	5	24	high
Seafood sticks	**12**	1 stick	2	1	trace	0
Seakale, steamed or boiled	**24**	3 heaped tbsp	2	1	1	med
Seaweed	**4**	2 tbsp	trace	1	trace	low
Seaweed, deep-fried	**131**	3 heaped tbsp	12	3	12	med
Seed cake	**423**	1 slice	6	58	20	low
Semolina (cream of wheat), canned	**172**	½ large can	3	27	5	low
Semolina, made with semi-skimmed milk	**150**	1 serving	6	29	2	low
Semolina, made with skimmed milk	**134**	1 serving	6	29	trace	low
Sesame seeds	**90**	1 tbsp	3	trace	9	high
Seven-up	**88**	1 tumbler	0	22	0	0
Seven-up, diet	**3**	1 tumbler	0	0	0	0
Seviche	**193**	1 serving	20	3	18	low
Shandy	**48**	1 tumbler	trace	13	trace	0
Shark steak, fried (sautéed)	**283**	1 steak	32	0	13	0
Shark steak, grilled (broiled)	**260**	1 steak	32	0	8	0

Food	kCal per portion	Portion size	Protein g	Carbs g	Fat g	Fibre
Shark's fin soup	99	2 ladlefuls	7	8	7	0
Sheep's milk	285	300 ml/½ pt/ 1¼ cups	16	15	18	0
Shepherd's pie	330	1 serving	24	25	19	med
Sherbet dip	78	1 small packet	0	19	0	0
Sherbet drink	91	1 tumbler	trace	20	1	0
Sherbet fountain	88	1 tube	trace	21	0	0
Sherbet lemons	20	1 sweet (candy)	0	5	0	0
Sherbet oranges	20	1 sweet (candy)	0	5	0	0
Sherbert pips	4	1 pip	0	1	0	0
Sherried chicken	197	¼ small chicken	29	7	4	low
Sherry, dry (fino)	58	1 double measure	trace	1	0	0
Sherry, medium (amontillado)	59	1 double measure	trace	2	0	0
Sherry, sweet (oloroso)	68	1 double measure	trace	3	0	0
Shiitake mushrooms, fresh, fried (sautéed)	50	2 tbsp	1	6	5	low
Shiitake mushrooms, fresh, stewed	27	2 tbsp	1	6	trace	low
Shiitake mushrooms, reconstituted dried, stewed	35	1 tbsp	1	7	trace	low
Shish kebabs	176	1 kebab	25	0	8	0
Shortbread fingers	67	1 finger	1	8	3	low
Shortcake biscuits (cookies)	43	1 biscuit	trace	6	2	low

Food	kCal per portion	Portion size	Protein g	Carbs g	Fat g	Fibre
Shredded wheat, dry	74	1 biscuit	2	15	trace	high
Shredded wheat, with semi-skimmed milk	205	2 biscuits	9	36	2	high
Shredded wheat, with skimmed milk	189	2 biscuits	9	36	1	high
Shredded wheat bitesize, dry	84	25 g/1 oz/½ cup	3	17	trace	high
Shredded wheat bitesize, with semi-skimmed milk	208	3 heaped tbsp	9	37	3	high
Shredded wheat bitesize, with skimmed milk	192	3 heaped tbsp	9	37	1	high
Shreddies, dry	86	25 g/1 oz/½ cup	2	18	trace	high
Shreddies, with semi-skimmed milk	213	5 heaped tbsp	9	38	3	high
Shreddies, with skimmed milk	197	5 heaped tbsp	9	38	1	high
Shreddies, chocolate, dry	91	25 g/1 oz/½ cup	2	20	trace	med
Shreddies, chocolate, with semi-skimmed milk	224	5 heaped tbsp	8	42	3	high
Shreddies, chocolate, with skimmed milk	208	5 heaped tbsp	8	42	1	high
Shreddies, frosted, dry	91	25 g/1 oz/½ cup	2	20	trace	high
Shreddies, frosted, with semi-skimmed milk	224	5 heaped tbsp	7	43	3	high
Shreddies, frosted, with skimmed milk	208	5 heaped tbsp	7	43	1	high

Food	kCal per portion	Portion size	Protein g	Carbs g	Fat g	Fibre
Shrimp *See* Prawns						
Shrimps, canned, drained	**80**	½ small can	18	0	trace	0
Shrimps, brown or pink, cooked, peeled	**15**	2 tbsp	8	0	trace	0
Shrimps, potted	**358**	1 small pot	16	0	32	0
Shropshire blue cheese	**87**	1 small wedge	5	trace	7	0
Sieved tomatoes *See* Passata						
Sild, in oil, drained	**108**	½ small can	12	0	7	0
Silverskin onions	**2**	1 onion	trace	trace	trace	low
Simnel cake	**298**	1 slice	4	49	11	med
Skate wings, in batter	**367**	1 wing	33	9	22	low
Skate wings, in black butter	**470**	1 wing	31	trace	41	0
Skippers, in oil, drained	**108**	½ small can	12	0	7	0
Skips	**87**	1 small packet	1	10	5	low
Slivovitz	**55**	1 single measure	trace	trace	0	0
Sloe gin	**35**	1 single measure	trace	8	0	0
Smacks, dry	**95**	25 g/1 oz/½ cup	2	21	trace	low
Smacks, with semi-skimmed milk	**209**	5 heaped tbsp	7	40	3	low
Smacks, with skimmed milk	**193**	5 heaped tbsp	7	40	1	low
Smarties (M&Ms)	**170**	1 tube	2	26	9	0
Smelts, fried (sautéed), in seasoned flour	**525**	5 fish	19	5	47	low

Food	kCal per portion	Portion size	Protein g	Carbs g	Fat g	Fibre
Smoked chicken breast	23	1 slice	2	trace	1	0
Smoked fish *See individual fish, e.g.* Salmon, smoked, *also* Smoked haddock *and* Smoked salmon						
Smoked haddock roulade	377	1 serving	30	16	20	low
Smoked pork ring	185	¼ ring	8	1	16	0
Smoked salmon	119	2 thin slices	21	0	4	0
Smoked salmon sandwiches	363	1 round	15	34	19	med
Smoked salmon and cream cheese bagel	353	1 bagel	17	44	12	med
Smoked salmon cream cheese sandwiches	429	1 round	15	34	26	med
Smoked salmon pâté	273	1 serving	10	0	26	0
Smoked turkey breast	21	1 slice	4	trace	trace	0
Snack shortcake	40	1 biscuit (cookie)	trace	5	2	low
Snack wafer bar	65	1 finger	trace	7	4	0
Snails, in garlic butter	311	6 snails	12	trace	25	low
Snapper, grilled (broiled)	218	1 medium fish	45	0	3	0
Snickers chocolate bar	329	1 standard bar	6	36	18	low
Snickers ice cream bar	230	1 standard bar	4	20	15	low
Snow peas *See Mangetout*						

Food	kCal per portion	Portion size	Protein g	Carbs g	Fat g	Fibre
Soba noodles, cooked	**228**	1 serving	11	48	trace	high
Soda bread, brown	**80**	1 thick slice	2	15	2	low
Soda bread, white	**82**	1 thick slice	2	12	2	low
Softgrain bread See Bread						
Sole See individual varieties, and cooking methods, e.g. Dover sole, Sole meunière, etc.						
Sole meunière	**376**	1 medium fish	44	trace	22	0
Sole mornay	**243**	1 fillet	47	7	12	low
Sole véronique	**184**	1 fillet	41	11	6	low
Solero ice lolly	**130**	1 lolly	2	20	4	0
Somen noodles, boiled	**230**	1 serving	7	48	trace	med
Soufflé See individual flavours, e.g. Cheese soufflé						
Soufflé omelette, savoury	**256**	2 eggs	14	trace	22	0
Soufflé omelette, sweet	**374**	2 eggs	14	10	22	0
Soupe au pistou, canned	**60**	2 ladlefuls	2	13	1	med
Soured (dairy sour) cream and chive dressing	**38**	1 tbsp	trace	trace	3	low
Soused herring	**180**	1 roll	12	6	12	0
Soused mackerel	**165**	1 roll	16	6	9	0

Food	kCal per portion	Portion size	Protein g	Carbs g	Fat g	Fibre
Southern comfort	70	1 single measure	trace	4	0	0
Southern fried chicken	494	2 pieces	36	19	29	low
Soy sauce	10	1 tsp	1	1	0	0
Soya beans, canned, drained	140	3 heaped tbsp	13	5	7	high
Soya beans, dried, soaked and cooked	141	3 heaped tbsp	14	5	7	high
Soya cheese	106	1 small wedge	6	trace	9	0
Soya cream substitute	28	1 tbsp	trace	1	3	low
Soya desserts, all flavours	103 (avge)	1 individual pot	3	19	2	low
Soya ice desserts, all flavours	44 (avge)	1 scoop	trace	5	2	low
Soya milk, sweetened	120	300 ml/½ pt/ 1¼ cups	9	12	5	low
Soya milk, unsweetened	96	300 ml/½ pt/ 1¼ cups	9	2	6	low
Soya yoghurt	90	1 individual pot	6	5	5	low
Spaghetti, dried, boiled	239	1 serving	8	51	2	med
Spaghetti, dried, wholemeal, boiled	259	1 serving	31	152	6	high
Spaghetti, fresh, boiled	301	1 serving	11	57	2	med
Spaghetti, with clams	433	1 serving	36	52	6	med
Spaghetti, with meatballs	718	1 serving	36	80	31	med

Food	kCal per portion	Portion size	Protein g	Carbs g	Fat g	Fibre
Spaghetti, with sausages in tomato sauce, canned	**116**	1 small can	8	25	9	med
Spaghetti, with tomato sauce	**432**	1 serving	12	71	13	high
Spaghetti, with tomato sauce, canned	**128**	1 small can	4	27	1	med
Spaghetti, with tomato sauce, no-added-sugar, canned	**101**	1 small can	4	20	1	med
Spaghetti alfredo	**478**	1 serving	23	67	13	high
Spaghetti bolognese	**456**	1 serving	20	56	19	med
Spaghetti carbonara	**402**	1 serving	10	56	22	med
Spaghetti hoops, canned	**122**	1 small can	4	26	1	med
Spaghetti hoops with hot dogs, canned	**180**	1 small can	6	22	8	low
Spaghetti napoletana	**432**	1 serving	12	71	13	high
Spam	**86**	1 slice	4	trace	8	0
Spanish omelette	**328**	2 eggs	16	17	22	med
Spanish rice	**228**	1 serving	6	46	2	high
Spare ribs See Pork spare ribs						
Special fried rice	**362**	1 serving	17	54	9	high
Special K, dry	**92**	25 g/1 oz/½ cup	4	18	trace	low
Special K, with semi-skimmed milk	**205**	5 heaped tbsp	10	36	trace	low

Food	kCal per portion	Portion size	Protein g	Carbs g	Fat g	Fibre
Special K, with skimmed milk	189	5 heaped tbsp	10	36	trace	low
Special K red berries, dry	92	25 g/1 oz/½ cup	3	18	trace	low
Special K red berries, with semi-skimmed milk	205	5 heaped tbsp	10	36	2	low
Special K red berries, with skimmed milk	189	5 heaped tbsp	10	36	trace	low
Spinach	12	1 good handful	1	1	trace	med
Spinach, cooked	19	3 heaped tbsp	2	1	1	med
Spinach, frozen, cooked	21	3 heaped tbsp	3	trace	1	med
Spinach and bacon salad	451	1 serving	18	9	44	med
Spinach roulade	327	1 serving	21	16	20	high
Spinach soup, home-made	132	2 ladlefuls	4	31	trace	med
Spirali (pasta shapes), dried, boiled	198	1 serving	7	42	1	med
Spirali, fresh, boiled	235	1 serving	9	45	2	med
Split pea soup, canned	142	1 serving	8	24	2	high
Split ice lolly, any flavour	83	1 lolly	1	13	3	0
Sponge cake	229	1 slice	3	26	13	low
Sponge cake, fatless	147	1 slice	5	26	3	low
Sponge cake, fatless, filled with cream	343	1 slice	5	36	22	low

Food	kCal per portion	Portion size	Protein g	Carbs g	Fat g	Fibre
Sponge cake, fatless, filled with jam (conserve)	**181**	1 slice	5	38	3	low
Sponge cake, victoria, filled with cream	**490**	1 slice	4	52	31	low
Sponge cake, victoria, filled with jam (conserve)	**302**	1 slice	4	64	5	low
Sponge (lady) fingers	**40**	1 finger	1	6	1	low
Sporties, dry	**89**	25 g/1 oz/½ cup	2	19	trace	high
Sporties, with semi-skimmed milk	**203**	5 heaped tbsp	8	37	3	high
Sporties, with skimmed milk	**187**	5 heaped tbsp	8	37	1	high
Spotted dick	**350**	1 serving	7	52	16	med
Sprats, fried (sautéed)	**393**	5 fish	14	4	35	low
Spring greens (collard greens), steamed or boiled	**20**	3 heaped tbsp	2	2	1	med
Spring onions (scallions)	**3**	1 onion	trace	trace	trace	low
Spring roll, large	**217**	1 large roll	7	21	12	low
Spring roll, small	**70**	1 small roll	3	7	3	low
Spring vegetable soup, canned	**62**	2 ladlefuls	2	13	trace	med
Spring vegetable soup, packet	**80**	2 ladlefuls	2	9	4	low
Sprite	**85**	1 tumbler	0	22	0	0
Sprite, diet	**5**	1 tumbler	0	0	0	0

Food	kCal per portion	Portion size	Protein g	Carbs g	Fat g	Fibre
Squab, roast	**303**	1 bird	37	0	18	0
Squab pie	**470**	1 serving	40	21	28	med
Squash *See* Marrow						
Squash, butternut	**9**	½ medium squash	trace	2	trace	low
Squash, fruit, diluted *See individual flavours, e.g.* Orange squash						
Squid, stewed in olive oil	**336**	1 serving	13	0	31	0
Squid, stuffed	**85**	1 squid	6	4	10	low
Squid rings, fried (sautéed), in batter	**235**	1 serving	14	19	12	low
Squid risotto	**369**	1 serving	9	52	15	low
Starfruit	**30**	1 fruit	trace	7	trace	med
Starburst sweets (candies)	**185**	1 tube	trace	38	3	0
Start, dry	**90**	25 g/1 oz/½ cup	2	20	trace	med
Start, with semi-skimmed milk	**201**	5 heaped tbsp	7	38	3	med
Start, with skimmed milk	**185**	5 heaped tbsp	7	38	1	med
Steak, fillet, fried (sautéed)	**359**	1 fillet	48	0	21	0
Steak, fillet, grilled (broiled)	**336**	1 fillet	48	0	16	0
Steak, rump or sirloin, fried	**430**	1 steak	50	0	25	0
Steak, rump or sirloin, grilled	**381**	1 steak	48	0	21	0

Food	kCal per portion	Portion size	Protein g	Carbs g	Fat g	Fibre
Steak and kidney pie	**500**	1 serving	26	28	32	med
Steak and kidney pie, individual	**484**	1 pie	13	38	31	med
Steak and kidney pudding	**431**	1 serving	34	24	23	low
Steak and onions	**463**	1 steak	49	8	27	med
Steak au poivre	**455**	1 steak	48	1	29	0
Steak chasseur	**417**	1 steak	49	7	21	0
Steak diane	**488**	1 steak	51	3	28	low
Steak sandwiches	**685**	1 round	53	34	38	low
Steamed sponge pudding	**340**	1 serving	6	45	16	med
Steamed suet pudding	**221**	1 serving	3	34	12	low
Stem lettuce See Chinese leaves						
Sticky toffee pudding	**313**	1 serving	3	47	12	low
Stifado	**565**	1 serving	45	6	16	med
Stilton cheese, blue	**103**	1 small wedge	6	trace	9	0
Stilton cheese, white	**94**	1 small wedge	6	trace	8	0
Stock cube, chicken	**32**	1 cube	1	3	2	0
Stock cube, meat	**32**	1 cube	1	2	2	0
Stock cube, vegetable	**33**	1 cube	1	3	2	0
Stollen	**177**	1 slice	2	26	13	med
Stout	**117**	1 small	1	6	trace	0
Straw mushrooms, canned, drained	**7**	¼ medium can	1	1	trace	0

Food	kCal per portion	Portion size	Protein g	Carbs g	Fat g	Fibre
Strawberries	27	3 heaped tbsp	1	6	trace	med
Strawberries, canned in natural juice	48	3 heaped tbsp	trace	13	trace	med
Strawberries, canned in syrup	65	3 heaped tbsp	trace	17	trace	med
Strawberry cheesecake	296	1 slice	5	32	17	low
Strawberry dessert	101	1 small pot	3	16	3	0
Strawberry ice cream	89	1 scoop	1	12	4	0
Strawberry milkshake, made with granules and semi-skimmed milk	138	1 tumbler	6	23	3	low
Strawberry jam (conserve)	39	1 tbsp	trace	10	0	0
Strawberry mousse	137	1 serving	4	18	6	low
Strawberry pavlova	320	1 serving	5	45	14	med
Strawberry shortcake	265	1 serving	5	35	12	low
Strawberry sorbet	57	1 scoop	trace	19	trace	low
Strawberry soufflé	325	1 serving	6	21	41	low
Streusel cake	157	1 slice	3	35	1	low
Striped bass, grilled (broiled)	153	1 piece of fillet	28	0	4	0
Stufato (Italian beef stew)	565	1 serving	45	6	16	med
Stuffing, made with breadcrumbs and herbs	14	1 tbsp	trace	3	trace	low
Stuffing, made with rice	31	1 tbsp	trace	5	1	low

Food	kCal per portion	Portion size	Protein g	Carbs g	Fat g	Fibre
Sugar puffs, dry	**97**	25 g/1 oz/½ cup	2	22	trace	low
Sugar puffs, with semi-skimmed milk	**212**	5 heaped tbsp	7	41	2	low
Sugar puffs, with skimmed milk	**196**	5 heaped tbsp	7	41	trace	low
Sugar snap peas	**57**	10 pods	5	8	1	high
Sugar snap peas, steamed or boiled	**52**	3 heaped tbsp	5	7	1	high
Sugar, all types	**20**	1 tsp	trace	5	trace	0
Sukiyaki	**246**	1 serving	20	20	9	high
Sultana bran, dry	**80**	25 g/1 oz/½ cup	2	16	trace	high
Sultana bran, with semi-skimmed milk	**185**	5 heaped tbsp	8	33	3	high
Sultana bran, with skimmed milk	**169**	5 heaped tbsp	8	33	1	high
Sultana (golden raisin) cake	**180**	1 slice	2	29	6	med
Sultanas (golden raisins)	**41**	1 small handful	trace	10	trace	high
Summer pudding	**266**	1 serving	7	59	1	high
Sunflower seeds	**87**	1 tbsp	4	2	7	high
Supernoodles, all flavours	**523** (avge)	1 packet	9	67	24	high
Surf 'n' turf	**516**	1 steak plus 2 breaded prawns (shrimp)	51	17	32	low
Sushi, mixed, average	**40**	1 piece	1	8	1	low
Sussex pond pudding	**391**	1 serving	3	50	24	low

Food	kCal per portion	Portion size	Protein g	Carbs g	Fat g	Fibre
Sustain, dry	90	25 g/1 oz/½ cup	2	18	1	med
Sustain, with semi-skimmed milk	201	5 heaped tbsp	8	36	3	med
Sustain, with skimmed milk	185	5 heaped tbsp	8	36	1	med
Swede (rutabaga), steamed or boiled	11	3 heaped tbsp	trace	2	trace	low
Sweet and sour chicken	165	1 serving	6	32	2	high
Sweet and sour pork	303	1 serving	26	31	9	med
Sweet and sour sauce	112	5 tbsp	trace	16	trace	low
Sweet potatoes, roasted	190	4 pieces	2	20	12	med
Sweet potatoes, steamed or boiled, mashed	84	3 heaped tbsp	1	20	trace	med
Sweetcorn (corn), kernels, canned	122	3 heaped tbsp	3	27	1	med
Sweetcorn, on the cob	99	1 cob	4	17	2	med
See also Corn cobs *and* Corn on the cob						
Swiss chard, steamed or boiled	25	3 heaped tbsp	2	4	trace	med
Swiss cheese *See also* Emmental *and* Gruyère	107	1 small wedge	8	1	8	0
Swiss cheese fondue	492	1 serving	30	8	29	0
Swiss cheese fondue, with French bread	762	1 serving plus 10 cubes of bread	40	62	31	med
Swiss (jelly) roll, chocolate	85	1 individual roll	3	14	3	low

Food	kCal per portion	Portion size	Protein g	Carbs g	Fat g	Fibre
Swiss roll, with jam (conserve)	**105**	1 individual roll	1	24	1	low
Swiss–style muesli *See* Muesli						
Swordfish steak, fried (sautéed)	**294**	1 steak	44	0	14	0
Swordfish steak, grilled (broiled)	**271**	1 steak	44	0	9	0
Syllabub	**428**	1 serving	1	5	35	0
Syrup, golden (light corn)	**45**	1 tbsp	trace	12	0	0
Syrup sauce, for ice cream, bottled, all flavours	**92** (avge)	2 tbsp	trace	23	0	0
Syrup sponge pudding	**369**	1 serving	6	53	16	med
Syrup tart	**368**	1 slice	4	60	14	med

Food	kCal per portion	Portion size	Protein g	Carbs g	Fat g	Fibre
Tabbouleh	278	3 heaped tbsp	7	41	10	high
Taco shell	57	1 shell	1	6	3	low
Taco shell, filled with chilli and salad	170	1 shell	7	12	10	med
Tagliarini (pasta strands), dried, boiled	239	1 serving	8	51	2	med
Tagliarini, fresh, boiled	301	1 serving	11	57	2	med
Tagliatelle (pasta ribbons), dried, boiled	239	1 serving	8	51	2	med
Tagliatelle, fresh, boiled	301	1 serving	11	57	2	med
Tahini paste	91	1 tbsp	3	trace	9	med
Tandoori chicken	750	½ small chicken	95	7	38	low
Tangerine	44	1 fruit	1	11	trace	med
Tangle twister ice lolly	90	1 lolly	1	18	2	low
Tango, lemon	98	1 tumbler	trace	23	trace	0
See also Apple tango, etc.						
Tango, orange	92	1 tumbler	0	25	0	0
Tapioca pudding, canned	169	½ large can	3	27	5	low
Tapioca pudding, made with semi-skimmed milk	150	1 serving	6	29	2	low
Tapioca pudding, made with skimmed milk	134	1 serving	6	29	trace	low
Taramasalata	223	2 tbsp	2	2	23	low
Tartare sauce	43	1 tbsp	trace	3	3	low

Food	kCal per portion	Portion size	Protein g	Carbs g	Fat g	Fibre
Taxi chocolate bar	**134**	1 standard bar	1	17	7	low
Tea, black	**0**	1 cup	trace	trace	trace	0
Tea, with lemon	**0**	1 cup	trace	trace	trace	0
Tea, with lemon and sugar	**20**	1 cup plus 1 spoonful of sugar	trace	5	trace	0
Tea, with milk	**7**	1 cup	trace	trace	1	0
Teacake	**180**	1 individual teacake	5	32	4	low
Teacake, toasted, with butter	**254**	1 individual teacake	5	32	12	low
Teacake, toasted, with low-fat spread	**219**	1 individual teacake	6	32	8	low
Tempura	**328**	1 serving	23	40	8	low
Tequila	**55**	1 single measure	trace	trace	0	0
Tequila sunrise	**232**	1 cocktail	1	24	trace	0
Teriyaki sauce	**14**	1 tbsp	trace	3	trace	low
Thai chicken, with noodles	**506**	1 serving	34	59	15	high
Thai chicken soup	**111**	2 ladlefuls	3	21	1	low
Thai fragrant rice, steamed or boiled	**248**	1 serving	3	56	2	low
Thai green chicken curry	**331**	1 serving	37	6	23	low
Thai red beef curry	**602**	1 serving	36	6	49	low
Thousand island dressing	**59**	1 tbsp	trace	2	5	low

Food	kCal per portion	Portion size	Protein g	Carbs g	Fat g	Fibre
Thousand island dressing, low-calorie	**12**	1 tbsp	trace	1	1	low
Tia maria	**79**	1 single measure	trace	6	0	0
Tilsit cheese	**96**	1 small wedge	7	trace	7	0
Time out chocolate bar	**105**	1 finger	1	6	6	low
Tip top topping	**16**	1 tbsp	1	1	1	low
Tipsy cake	**488**	1 slice	5	41	32	low
Tiramisu	**222**	1 serving	6	24	11	low
Tisanes, all flavours	**0**	1 cup	trace	trace	trace	0
Tizer	**82**	1 tumbler	0	20	trace	low
Tizer, diet	**0**	1 tumbler	0	trace	trace	low
Toad-in-the-hole	**462**	2 thick sausages plus batter	17	33	30	med
Toast, white, with butter	**155**	1 medium slice	3	18	9	low
Toast, white, with low-fat spread	**120**	1 medium slice	4	18	5	low
Toast, wholemeal, with butter	**153**	1 medium slice	3	15	10	high
Toast, wholemeal, with low-fat spread	**118**	1 medium slice	4	15	6	high
Toasted cheese and ham sandwiches	**438**	1 round	20	36	27	med
Toffee bon bons	**29**	1 toffee	0	6	1	0
Toffee apple	**251**	1 apple	4	66	trace	high
Toffee crisp chocolate bar	**237**	1 standard bar	2	30	12	low

Food	kCal per portion	Portion size	Protein g	Carbs g	Fat g	Fibre
Toffee fudge ice cream	**90**	1 scoop	1	12	4	0
Toffees, mixed	**20**	1 toffee	trace	1	0	0
Toffos, assorted	**203**	1 tube	1	31	8	0
Tofu, firm	**62**	½ block	8	2	2	low
Tofu, fried (sautéed)	**308**	½ block	20	12	24	med
Tofu, marinated, baked	**139**	½ block	12	4	10	med
Tofu, silken	**55**	½ block	5	2	2	low
Tofu, smoked	**148**	½ block	36	1	9	low
Tofu and vegetable stir-fry	**334**	1 serving	17	24	21	high
Tofu burger	**154**	1 burger	10	6	12	med
Tomato	**13**	1 fruit	1	2	trace	low
Tomato, stuffed, baked	**53**	1 large	3	9	1	med
Tomato and herb pasta sauce, ready-made	**79**	¼ jar	1	16	trace	low
Tomato and lentil soup, canned	**108**	2 ladlefuls	6	20	trace	med
Tomato and lentil soup, home-made	**188**	2 ladlefuls	8	26	8	med
Tomato and lentil soup, instant	**73**	1 mug	3	15	1	low
Tomato and onion salad	**35**	1 serving	2	11	trace	med
Tomato and onion salad, dressed	**132**	1 serving	2	11	17	med
Tomato and orange soup, canned	**80**	2 ladlefuls	2	17	1	low

Food	kCal per portion	Portion size	Protein g	Carbs g	Fat g	Fibre
Tomato and orange soup, home-made	103	2 ladlefuls	2	15	4	med
Tomato and rice soup, canned	94	2 ladlefuls	2	17	2	low
Tomato chutney	24	1 tbsp	trace	6	trace	low
Tomato juice	28	1 tumbler	2	6	trace	low
Tomato juice cocktail	36	1 tumbler	2	19	0	low
Tomato ketchup (catsup)	15	1 tbsp	trace	4	trace	low
Tomato relish	16	1 tbsp	trace	3	trace	low
Tomato risotto	403	1 serving	7	58	18	med
Tomato sauce, home-made	67	5 tbsp	2	6	4	med
Tomato soup, cream of, canned	110	2 ladlefuls	2	12	7	low
Tomato soup, home-made	86	2 ladlefuls	3	11	4	low
Tomato soup, instant	85	1 mug	1	17	2	med
Tomato soup, low-fat, canned	50	2 ladlefuls	1	8	1	low
Tomatoes, canned	32	1 small can	2	6	trace	med
Tomatoes, fried (sautéed)	68	2 halves	trace	4	6	low
Tomatoes, grilled (broiled)	37	2 halves	1	7	1	low
Tomatoes, sieved	29	5 tbsp	1	6	trace	0
Tomatoes, stewed	25	2 whole	1	4	trace	med
Tomatoes, sun-dried	5	1 piece	trace	1	trace	low

Food	kCal per portion	Portion size	Protein g	Carbs g	Fat g	Fibre
Tomatoes, sun-dried, in oil, drained	7	1 piece	trace	1	1	low
Tongue, lunch	43	1 slice	1	0	3	0
Tongue, ox, pressed and sliced	73	1 slice	5	0	6	0
Tongue, pork, pressed and sliced	47	1 slice	1	0	4	0
Tongues, lambs', canned	213	½ medium can	16	0	16	0
Tonic water	43	1 tumbler	0	10	0	0
Tonic water, low-calorie	4	1 tumbler	trace	0	0	0
Topic chocolate bar	233	1 standard bar	3	27	12	low
Tornado ice cream	61	1 ice	0	15	0	0
Tortellini (stuffed pasta), dried, boiled	291	1 serving	9	45	6	med
Tortellini, fresh, boiled	229	1 serving	9	40	4	med
Tortilla (spanish omelette)	328	2 eggs	16	17	22	med
Tortilla chips, all flavours	229	1 small bag	4	30	11	med
Tortillas, corn	58	1 medium tortilla	1	12	1	med
Tortillas, flour	159	1 medium tortilla	4	27	3	med
Tournedos rossini	477	1 fillet steak	52	9	25	low
Tracker bars, all flavours	192 (avge)	1 standard bar	3	22	10	med
Treacle, black (molasses)	38	1 tbsp	trace	10	0	0
Treacle pudding	369	1 serving	6	53	16	med
Treacle tart	368	1 slice	4	60	14	med

Food	kCal per portion	Portion size	Protein g	Carbs g	Fat g	Fibre
Treacle toffee	20	1 piece	trace	1	0	0
Trifle	372	1 serving	10	69	6	high
Trinity cream	453	1 serving	1	15	50	0
Trio chocolate bar	111	1 standard bar	1	12	6	low
Triple chocolate bar	99	1 standard bar	1	12	5	low
Tropical fruit salad	86	3 heaped tbsp	trace	22	trace	med
Trout, baked, stuffed	326	1 medium fish	56	41	39	med
Trout, fried (sautéed)	232	1 medium fish	33	0	13	0
Trout, grilled (broiled)	209	1 medium fish	33	0	8	0
Trout, poached or steamed	200	1 medium fish	35	0	7	0
Trout, smoked	136	1 fillet	23	0	5	0
Trout, smoked, pâté	269	1 serving	11	0	24	0
Trout meunière	388	1 medium fish	46	trace	29	0
Trout with almonds	464	1 medium fish	48	1	36	med
Truffles, chocolate	50	1 truffle	1	6	2	low
Truite au bleu	200	1 medium fish	35	0	7	0
Tuc crackers	25	1 cracker	trace	3	1	low
Tuc savoury sandwiches	76	1 sandwich	1	7	5	low
Tuna, canned in brine, drained	107	½ standard can	23	0	trace	0
Tuna, canned in oil, drained	182	½ standard can	27	0	7	0
Tuna and cucumber sandwiches	352	1 round	15	35	18	med

Food	kCal per portion	Portion size	Protein g	Carbs g	Fat g	Fibre
Tuna and pasta casserole	285	1 serving	22	30	9	med
Tuna and sweetcorn pasta	451	1 serving	37	50	11	med
Tuna mornay	241	1 serving	29	7	10	low
Tuna mousse	185	1 serving	11	6	10	low
Tuna salad	138	1 serving	25	5	1	high
Tuna salad, with mayonnaise	344	1 serving	25	11	23	high
Tuna steak, fried (sautéed)	345	1 steak	52	0	15	0
Tuna steak, grilled (broiled)	322	1 steak	52	0	10	0
Tunes sweets (candies)	145	1 tube	0	36	0	0
Turbot, grilled (broiled)	194	1 piece of fillet	33	0	6	0
Turbot, steamed or poached	159	1 piece of fillet	36	0	1	0
Turkey, breast, smoked	21	1 slice	4	trace	trace	0
Turkey, fillets, fried (sautéed)	248	1 medium fillet	40	0	9	0
Turkey fillets, grilled (broiled)	225	1 medium fillet	40	0	4	0
Turkey fillets, fried, in breadcrumbs	326	1 medium fillet	43	13	9	low
Turkey, minced (ground), stewed	197	1 serving	31	0	5	0
Turkey, roast, with skin	171	2 medium slices	28	0	6	0
Turkey, roast, without skin	140	2 medium slices	29	0	3	0

Food	kCal per portion	Portion size	Protein g	Carbs g	Fat g	Fibre
Turkey, roast, with stuffing and sausagemeat	229	1 serving	33	12	5	med
Turkey and vegetable casserole	298	1 serving	23	32	8	med
Turkey and vegetable soup, home-made	134	2 ladlefuls	10	14	4	med
Turkey and vegetable stir-fry	259	1 serving	29	31	3	high
Turkey bacon, grilled (broiled)	34	1 slice	2	trace	3	0
Turkey burger in a bun, with relish, home-made	357	1 burger in a bun	38	32	9	low
Turkey fingers, fried (sautéed), in batter or breadcrumbs	178	1 finger	9	11	11	low
Turkey ham	36	1 slice	5	trace	1	0
Turkey pot pie	485	1 slice	17	28	39	low
Turkey roll	41	1 slice	5	trace	2	0
Turkey sandwiches	345	1 round	10	34	19	med
Turkey soup, home-made	111	2 ladlefuls	13	7	2	0
Turkey stew	430	1 serving	34	65	3	med
Turkish delight, chocolate covered	185	1 standard bar	1	37	4	0
Turkish delight, in icing (confectioners') sugar	29	1 cube	trace	8	0	0
Turnips, glazed	55	3 heaped tbsp	1	15	trace	med

Food	kCal per portion	Portion size	Protein g	Carbs g	Fat g	Fibre
Turnips, steamed or boiled	**12**	3 heaped tbsp	1	2	trace	med
Tuscan bean salad	**120**	3 heaped tbsp	4	12	5	high
Tutti frutti ice cream	**75**	1 scoop	1	5	7	low
Twiglets	**136**	1 small bag	4	16	3	med
Twirl chocolate bar	**115**	1 finger	2	12	7	0
Twistetti (pasta shapes), dried, boiled	**198**	1 serving	7	42	1	med
Twistetti, fresh, boiled	**235**	1 serving	9	45	2	med
Twix chocolate bar	**143**	1 finger	2	18	7	low
Twix ice cream	228	1 standard bar	3	23	14	low
Tzatziki	**20**	2 tbsp	1	1	1	low

Food	kCal per portion	Portion size	Protein g	Carbs g	Fat g	Fibre
Vacherin, with cream and fruit	320	1 slice	5	45	14	med
Vanilla fudge	77	1 square	trace	14	2	0
Vanilla cheesecake	490	1 slice	4	30	27	low
Vanilla ice cream, dairy	97	1 scoop	2	12	5	0
Vanilla ice cream, non-dairy	89	1 scoop	2	11	4	0
Vanilla soufflé	236	1 serving	7	26	1	low
Veal, cutlet, fried (sautéed), in breadcrumbs,	376	1 cutlet	55	8	14	low
Veal, cutlet, grilled (broiled)	300	1 cutlet	52	0	9	0
Veal, escalope, fried, in breadcrumbs	335	1 escalope	32	20	15	low
Veal, roast	230	2 thick slices	32	0	11	0
Veal birds	450	2 rolls	52	12	20	low
Veal fricassée	339	1 serving	27	34	9	low
Vegemite	8	1 tsp	1	trace	0	0
Vegetable bake	360	1 serving	12	33	10	high
Vegetable casserole	228	1 serving	12	33	6	high
Vegetable cottage pie	350	1 serving	15	48	12	high
Vegetable curry	183	1 serving	5	34	4	high
Vegetable deluxe burger	423	1 burger in a bun	10	54	18	high
Vegetable goulash	338	1 serving	12	142	15	high
Vegetable juice	41	1 tumbler	trace	9	trace	low

Food	kCal per portion	Portion size	Protein g	Carbs g	Fat g	Fibre
Vegetable lasagne	424	1 serving	15	50	10	high
Vegetable pâté	138	1 serving	10	1	10	low
Vegetable pie	425	1 individual pie	6	52	23	med
Vegetable risotto	372	1 serving	6	58	15	low
Vegetable samosa	236	1 samosa	1	11	21	med
Vegetable soup, canned	74	2 ladlefuls	3	13	1	high
Vegetable soup, home-made	93	2 ladlefuls	3	4	trace	high
Vegetable soup, packet	46	2 ladlefuls	2	8	1	low
Vegetable stew	186	1 serving	7	31	4	high
Vegetable stir-fry	169	1 serving	7	15	6	high
Vegetable terrine	155	1 thick slice	8	17	7	high
Vegetables, mixed, canned, drained	38	3 heaped tbsp	2	6	1	med
Vegetables, mixed, frozen, cooked	42	3 heaped tbsp	3	7	trace	high
Veggie burger	85	1 burger	7	5	4	med
Veggie sausage	75	1 sausage	3	6	4	med
Velouté sauce	99	5 tbsp	1	4	9	low
Venison, roast	198	2 thick slices	35	0	6	0
Venison, stewed	225	1 serving	25	8	7	low
Vermicelli (pasta strands), dried, boiled	239	1 serving	8	51	2	med
Vermicelli, fresh, boiled	301	1 serving	11	57	2	med

Food	kCal per portion	Portion size	Protein g	Carbs g	Fat g	Fibre
Vermouth, bianco	67	1 double measure	trace	8	0	0
Vermouth, extra dry	59	1 double measure	trace	3	0	0
Vermouth, red	75	1 double measure	trace	8	0	0
Vermouth, rosso	85	1 double measure	trace	8	0	0
Vichyssoise, canned	108	2 ladlefuls	2	12	6	low
Vichyssoise, home-made	117	2 ladlefuls	2	8	6	low
Victoria sandwich, filled with jam (conserve)	302	1 slice	4	64	5	low
Viennetta, all flavours	227 (avge)	1 slice	3	23	14	0
Vienna bread	109	1 thick slice	3	15	1	low
Viennese finger, filled	81	1 biscuit (cookie)	1	9	5	low
Vimto	52	1 tumbler	trace	20	trace	0
Vinaigrette dressing	101	1 tbsp	trace	trace	11	0
Vinaigrette dressing, low-calorie	5	1 tbsp	trace	1	trace	0
Vine leaves, stuffed	221	2 rolls	18	19	9	high
Vinegar, all types	1	1 tsp	trace	0	0	0
Vitbe bread	82	1 medium slice	3	16	1	med
Vitello tonnato	594	1 escalope	44	20	37	low
Vodka	55	1 single measure	trace	trace	0	0
Vodka and orange	108	1 single measure	trace	7	0	0
Vodka and tonic	76	1 single measure plus 1 mixer	trace	5	0	0
Vodka and tonic, low-calorie	58	1 single measure plus 1 mixer	trace	trace	trace	0

Food	kCal per portion	Portion size	Protein g	Carbs g	Fat g	Fibre
Vodka martini	**114**	1 cocktail	trace	3	trace	0
Vol-au-vents, all flavours	**286** (avge)	1 medium	11	20	18	low
Vol-au-vents, cocktail, all flavours	**143** (avge)	1 small	5	10	9	low

Food	kCal per portion	Portion size	Protein g	Carbs g	Fat g	Fibre
Wafer biscuits (cookies), chocolate-covered	115	1 biscuit	1	13	6	low
Wafer biscuits, filled	39	1 biscuit	1	7	2	low
Wafers, for ice cream	17	1 wafer	2	4	trace	low
Waffle, potato, fried (sautéed) or baked	84	1 waffle	1	13	3	low
Waffle, sweet	240	1 waffle	8	30	8	low
Waffles, sweet, with maple syrup	533	2 waffles	16	75	16	med
Waffles, with bacon and maple syrup	799	2 waffles plus 2 rashers (slices) of bacon	36	75	48	med
Walnut cake	344	1 slice	7	34	19	med
Walnut whip	165	1 whip	7	20	8	low
Walnut whirl, chocolate	20	1 chocolate	trace	2	1	low
Walnuts, shelled	172	25 g/1 oz/¼ cup	4	1	17	high
Water biscuits (crackers)	33	1 biscuit	1	6	1	low
Water chestnuts, canned, drained	14	4 pieces	trace	3	trace	low
Watercress	3	1 good handful	trace	trace	trace	med
Watercress soup	99	2 ladlefuls	1	14	2	low
Watermelon	66	1 large wedge	1	14	1	low
Weetabix, dry	64	1 biscuit	2	13	trace	high
Weetabix, with semi-skimmed milk	169	2 biscuits	8	32	trace	high
Weetabix, with skimmed milk	185	2 biscuits	8	32	2	high

Food	kCal per portion	Portion size	Protein g	Carbs g	Fat g	Fibre
Weetaflakes, dry	90	25 g/1 oz/½ cup	2	20	1	high
Weetaflakes, with semi skimmed milk-	201	5 heaped tbsp	8	38	3	high
Weetaflakes, with skimmed milk	185	5 heaped tbsp	8	38	1	high
Weetos, dry	96	25 g/1 oz/½ cup	1	20	1	med
Weetos, with semi-skimmed milk	172	5 heaped tbsp	6	30	4	med
Weetos, with skimmed milk	154	5 heaped tbsp	6	30	2	med
Welsh rarebit	242	1 slice	10	21	13	low
Wensleydale cheese	94	1 small wedge	6	trace	8	0
Westphalian ham	29	1 slice	4	trace	2	0
Wheat bran	31	1 tbsp	2	4	1	high
Wheat crunchies, all flavours	180 (avge)	1 small packet	4	20	9	low
Whelks, boiled	14	1 serving	3	trace	trace	0
Whippy ice cream	85	1 cornet	2	12	3	low
Whisky	55	1 single measure	trace	trace	0	0
Whisky and coke	99	1 single measure plus 1 mixer	trace	6	0	0
Whisky and coke, low-calorie	56	1 single measure plus 1 mixer	trace	trace	trace	0
Whisky and ginger ale	75	1 single measure plus 1 mixer	trace	5	0	0
Whisky and ginger ale, low-calorie	55	1 single measure plus 1 tumbler	trace	trace	0	0

Food	kCal per portion	Portion size	Protein g	Carbs g	Fat g	Fibre
Whisky mac	**255**	1 single measure plus 1 double measure	trace	trace	0	0
Whisky sour	**157**	1 cocktail	0	14	0	0
White pudding, fried (sautéed) or baked	**450**	2 thick slices	7	36	32	low
White sauce, savoury, made with semi-skimmed milk	**96**	5 tbsp	3	8	6	low
White sauce, savoury, made with skimmed milk	**86**	5 tbsp	3	8	5	low
White sauce, sweet, made with semi-skimmed milk	**112**	5 tbsp	3	14	5	low
White sauce, sweet, made with skimmed milk	**92**	5 tbsp	3	14	4	low
White stilton cheese	**94**	1 small wedge	6	trace	8	0
White wine sauce	**75**	5 tbsp	2	6	2	low
Whitebait, fried (sautéed)	**525**	1 serving	19	5	47	low
Whiting, fried (sautéed), in breadcrumbs	**334**	1 fillet	31	12	17	low
Whiting, poached or steamed	**110**	1 fillet	24	0	1	0
Whiting, smoked, poached	**166**	1 fillet	25	1	1	0
Wholegrain mustard	**7**	1 tsp	2	1	trace	low
Wholenut chocolate bar	**270**	1 standard bar	5	24	17	med

Food	kCal per portion	Portion size	Protein g	Carbs g	Fat g	Fibre
Whopper	660	1 burger	29	47	40	high
Whopper, with cheese	760	1 burger	35	47	48	high
Whopper, double	920	2 burgers	49	47	21	high
Whopper, double, with cheese	1010	2 burgers	55	47	67	high
Wiener schnitzel	335	1 schnitzel	32	20	15	low
Wild rice, cooked	182	1 serving	7	6	trace	0
Wild rice mix, cooked	177	1 serving	6	31	1	low
Winders, real fruit	55	1 roll	trace	11	1	low
Wine gums	119	1 tube	3	27	trace	0
Wine, dry white, sparkling	95	1 wine glass	trace	2	0	0
Wine, dry white	82	1 wine glass	trace	1	0	0
Wine, low-alcohol, red	70	1 wine glass	trace	2	0	0
Wine, low-alcohol, rosé	70	1 wine glass	trace	2	0	0
Wine, low-alcohol, white	70	1 wine glass	trace	2	0	0
Wine, medium white	94	1 wine glass	trace	4	0	0
Wine, mulled	105	1 wine glass	trace	5	0	0
Wine, red	85	1 wine glass	trace	trace	trace	0
Wine, rosé	89	1 wine glass	trace	1	0	0
Wine, sweet	117	1 wine glass	trace	7	0	0
Winkles	14	1 serving	3	trace	trace	0
Winter radish	12	1 radish	1	2	trace	low
Wispa chocolate bar	210	1 standard bar	3	21	13	0
Wispa, gold	265	1 standard bar	3	29	15	0

Food	kCal per portion	Portion size	Protein g	Carbs g	Fat g	Fibre
Wispa, mint	**275**	1 standard bar	3	27	17	0
Witch, fried (sautéed), in breadcrumbs	**342**	1 medium fish	25	15	21	low
Witch, grilled (broiled)	**158**	1 medium fish	25	0	4	0
Witch, poached or steamed	**112**	1 medium fish	25	0	1	0
Woodcock, roast	**303**	1 bird	37	0	18	0
Worcestershire sauce	**17**	1 tbsp	trace	4	0	0
Wotsits, all flavours	**115** (avge)	1 small packet	2	12	7	low

Food	kCal per portion	Portion size	Protein g	Carbs g	Fat g	Fibre
Yam, roast	**156**	4 pieces	2	33	5	med
Yam, steamed or boiled, mashed	**133**	3 heaped tbsp	2	33	trace	med
Yeast extract	**9**	1 tsp	2	trace	trace	0
Yellow bean sauce	**19**	1 tbsp	trace	4	trace	low
Yellow beans, fresh, steamed or boiled	**25**	3 heaped tbsp	2	5	trace	high
Yellow melon	**63**	1 large wedge	1	15	trace	med
Yoghurt (plain)	**99**	1 individual pot	7	10	4	0
Yoghurt, all flavours	**131** (avge)	1 individual pot	6	20	4	0
Yoghurt, bio	**56**	1 small pot	5	7	1	0
Yoghurt, custard-style	**161**	1 small pot	8	3	13	0
Yoghurt, drinking	**124**	1 tumbler	6	26	trace	0
Yoghurt, fruit corner	**219**	1 individual carton	6	26	7	low
Yoghurt, greek-style, cows'	**161**	1 individual pot	8	3	13	0
Yoghurt, greek-style, sheep's	**149**	1 individual pot	6	8	10	0
Yoghurt, low-calorie	**51**	1 individual pot	5	7	trace	0
Yoghurt, low-fat, plain	**70**	1 individual pot	6	9	1	0
Yoghurt, low-fat, all flavours	**112** (avge)	1 individual pot	5	22	1	0
Yoghurt, soya	**90**	1 individual pot	6	5	5	0
Yoghurt ice-cream, all flavours	**53** (avge)	1 scoop	3	8	1	low

Food	kCal per portion	Portion size	Protein g	Carbs g	Fat g	Fibre
Yoghurt jelly (jello), made with plain, low-fat yoghurt	**60**	1 serving	5	12	1	0
Yorkie bar, milk	**317**	1 standard bar	4	35	18	0
Yorkie bar, nut	**312**	1 standard bar	6	26	10	low
Yorkie bar, raisin and biscuit (cookie)	**265**	1 standard bar	3	32	13	low
Yorkshire parkin	**185**	1 piece	2	29	7	low
Yorkshire pudding	**62**	1 small pudding	2	7	3	low

Food	kCal per portion	Portion size	Protein g	Carbs g	Fat g	Fibre
Zabaglione	**87**	1 serving	3	8	3	0
Zite (pasta shapes), dried, boiled	**198**	1 serving	7	42	1	med
Zite, fresh, boiled	**235**	1 serving	9	45	2	med
Zoom ice lolly	**46**	1 lolly	trace	10	trace	0
Zucchini *See* Courgettes						